ESSENTIAL GUIDE ON INSULIN RESISTANCE DIET TO HELP PEOPLE LOSE WEIGHT

———

Elena Miller

INSULIN RESISTANCE DIET

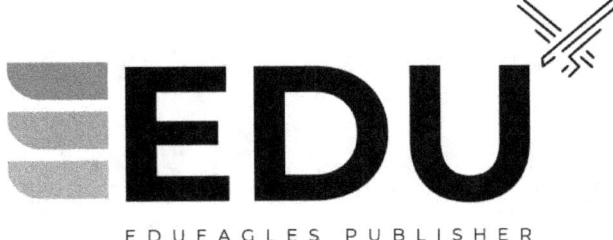

EDUEAGLES PUBLISHER

Table Of Contents

INTRODUCTION

Most cases of reactive hypoglycemia are labeled idiopathic, which means "unknown cause". I believe insulin resistance causes most cases of idiopathic reactive hypoglycemia, and that insulin resistance is caused, in turn, by diet and heredity. Insulin resistance can be an early warning sign of Type II diabetes and studies have shown that Type II diabetics may have been insulin resistant for up to 12 years before diagnosis.

By far the most common cases of chronic hypoglycemia are types of reactive hypoglycemia. Reactive hypoglycemia is also called postprandial hypoglycemia, postprandial syndrome or functional hypoglycemia and symptoms appear two to five hours after you eat. Postprandial, by the way, simply means, "after eating".)

Insulin is supposed to trigger the acceptance of circulating blood sugar (glucose) into the body's cells, but over time and with an over refined diet, your cells can become insulin resistant. When cells are insulin resistant, it takes increasing amounts of insulin to trigger the acceptance of additional sugar into cells in your body.

Unchecked, this often progresses to Type II diabetes when your pancreas just gives up after years of producing more insulin than it was meant to. Your blood pressure, cholesterol and tryglycerides readings go up, and you are now at risk of heart attack.

Syndrome X (aka Insulin Resistance Syndrome) is defined as insulin resistance with high blood pressure and high tryglycerides. If you have Syndrome X, you are also at increased risk of developing cancer.

As with almost everything, some people are more quickly affected by adverse conditions than others are. We already know that some people are more likely to get diabetes or cancer or heart disease. And this is at least partly because some people are more likely to have trouble with our over processed and over refined diet. This is the heredity component of insulin resistance. The more refined foods, especially sugar, that we eat, the more insulin the pancreas produces. No one should be eating the amounts of sugar that most of us do, but some people's bodies can resist the effects longer.

Insulin resistance happens when your body has been overwhelmed with too much insulin for so long that your cells stop listening. For the cells of your body, a constantly high level of insulin is just like constant noise in your ears.

Over time, you learn to ignore the noise, and it takes a

louder sound to get your attention. Your cells view insulin in the same way. It takes more and more insulin to get your cells to pay attention. When your cells ignore insulin and refuse to "open" to take in sugar from your blood, your pancreas simply sends more insulin until your cells begin to respond. The excess insulin has several effects. First, by the time the cells finally begin to accept sugar, there is so much insulin available that your blood sugar drops too much-hypoglycemia. Second, insulin resistance causes more insulin resistance, so eventually there is a lot of insulin floating around your system all the time.

All that insulin makes it difficult to keep your blood sugar steady. When the insulin resistance train has been accelerating on its track for a while, your body really isn't handling sugar properly anymore, and you will have an "abnormal sugar metabolism". One way an abnormal sugar metabolism will show up is in chronic hypoglycemia.

Processing sugar is hard work. Eating a donut or a cookie or a granola bar causes a blood sugar spike that the pancreas must deal with. Every spike requires the release of insulin to get it back under control. If we eat a lot of refined foods containing a lot of sugar, we find ourselves living on the blood sugar roller coaster. Abnormal sugar handling, over time, causes increased insulin resistance.

We know that a high level of sugar in the blood is bad.

That's why diabetics stop eating sweets and take medication. A high level of insulin is also bad, but more insidious. Insulin is not meant to sit around in the body all the time, and excess insulin causes a host of problems. For one thing, insulin is a storage hormone, so if you have too much insulin, you will gain weight because excess sugar is stored as fat.

Excess weight is a major risk factor for diabetes, and so is overworking the pancreas by producing too much insulin. In early Type II diabetes, the pancreas is working very hard to keep up with the demand. Insulin levels in the body are abnormally high, and your blood sugar may be alternating between high and low. This leads to full-blown diabetes when the over-worked pancreas simply can't produce the amounts of insulin needed to overcome the insulin resistance of the body's cells. This slide into Type II diabetes is much more likely in people who are significantly overweight. Sixty-five percent of people living with diabetes will die of a heart attack or stroke.

In addition to Type II diabetes, insulin resistance can cause an increase in blood pressure, "bad" cholesterol and tryglycerides. Dr. Gerald Reaven first recognized that these problems are linked in the late 1980s. He coined the term Syndrome X because no one knew at the time how these problems were linked or what caused them. But it is as clear now as it was then-this combination is a heart attack waiting to happen!

In this book, Syndrome X, Dr. Reaven states that Syndrome X "...may be the cause of 50 percent of all heart attacks". Dr. Reaven also suggests that Insulin Resistance Syndrome "...affects between 60-75 million Americans". More recently, experts have also come to believe that Syndrome X (aka insulin resistance syndrome) also increases the risk of cancer.

The more of the following risk factors you have, the greater the chance you have Syndrome X:

Overweight, a sedentary lifestyle, over age 40, non-Caucasian ethnicity, a family history of Type II diabetes, high blood pressure or cardiovascular disease, a history of glucose intolerance, a diagnosis of high blood pressure, elevated triglycerides/low HDL cholesterol, or cardiovascular disease.

This makes it very clear that whether or not you are hypoglycemic or have high blood sugar, you may be at risk if you have any of these risk factors. Consult your physician, and be prepared to change your diet and your lifestyle ASAP to turn back the advance of abnormal blood sugar, insulin resistance and Syndrome X!

WHAT IS INSULIN RESISTANCE?

When some cells of human body are unable to respond to insulin properly and completely, the cells are said to be affected by insulin resistance. This is a disease in which the human body is not able to take up the insulin properly and thus, glucose is not broken down in our body and the body does not deals with the sugar well. Since insulin is not taken up by the body, this may lead to the accumulation of a large amount of insulin in the blood, which further complexes the situation. This situation is known as hyperinsulinemia.

Various Causes of IR

The causes of "IR" could be many and it is difficult to be sure which one is applicable to which person. Generally, like many other diseases, this could also be passed over generations. It means that if any one of your family members have suffered from "IR" in the past, you are more likely to catch the disorder than the one who has no family history of "IR". Moreover, physical activity is important for avoiding this disease as this would make the cells more active. Obesity is yet another factor leading to insulin resistance in the body cells.

Problems Associated with IR

Obesity is the most visible effect of insulin resistance. Not only abdominal obesity, but a weight gain in general, all over your body, is observed, that too, at a rapid pace. Blood pressure going high and increased cholesterol level are another major problems associated with "IR". Diabetes is also caused by this disorder. And, last, but not the least, "IR" might add to the heart diseases as well. This means that cardio logical diseases can also be observed in the "IR" patients.

How to Manage IR?

Once you are diagnosed to be insulin resistant, it is very important to manage the disorder as carelessness might result in more dangerous outcomes and the conditions may worsen. There are generally two ways for managing insulin resistance, either you reduce the need of insulin, or, the second option; you may increase the response of body cells towards the insulin.

The most common thing that needs to be followed while curing or managing any health related disorder is to modify your life style. The diet is the most important factor. Including those food items which have low glycaemia index is necessary as it would require less insulin to absorb low level of glucose and hence less insulin needs to be secreted by the body. Further, since body weight is an important factor, in case you have high body weight and you are obese, you need to exercise a lot and include it in your daily lifestyle so that it becomes a habit and overweight could be managed.

As mentioned earlier, the people having genetic background of insulin resistance are more likely to suffer from the disorder; hence, they should take care of themselves more than the other people.

HOW TO AVOID INSULIN RESISTANCE AND MANAGE DIABETES - NATURALLY

Insulin resistance is when the cell (particularly liver, muscle and fat cells, with the liver losing sensitivity first, then the muscle and then the fat cells) loses its responsiveness on the insulin receptor site. Your body adds more and more insulin to store fat. Overtime, the pancreas give up leading to type II diabetes.

In type II diabetes, your body isn't making enough insulin and/or the cells are resistant to insulin causing too much sugar to remain in the blood.

Insulin is necessary for your body's use of sugar. Sugar is the basic fuel for your cells in the body, and insulin takes the sugar from the blood into the cells.

A fasting blood glucose level higher than 100-125 mg/dL is not indicative of diabetes, but it can be indicative of insulin resistance, and is above normal levels. Optimum serum glucose range is 80-95. Fasting serum insulin levels should be below 10.

Controlling your insulin levels with diet/nutrition, lifestyle modifications, exercise and supplements are a powerful anti-aging strategy and a must for health, vitality, longevity and fat loss.

Insulin Resistance Symptoms and Conditions:

- ✓ Brain fogginess and inability to focus
- ✓ Elevated triglycerides. Optimum range: 70-110 mg/dL. (40 to 60% of total cholesterol). This can only be determined with a fasting test. Triglycerides are a component of fat stored in the tissue. Decreased HDL with elevated triglycerides is a more significant indicator of risk to heart disease than total cholesterol over 200 mg/dL. Triglycerides are often increased with dysinsulinism (Syndrome-X/Metabolic Syndrome), alcoholism (GGT/GGTP also generally increased) and diabetes.
- ✓ Excess fat around your midsection or scapula area
- ✓ Hypertension
- ✓ Intestinal bloating
- ✓ Low HDL levels. Optimum range: Males - above 55 mg/dL. Females - above 60 mg/dL. Should be > than 25% of total cholesterol. Most effective way to > HDL is > exercise.
- ✓ Sleepiness and fatigue

Type II diabetes

When glucose (sugar) builds up in the blood instead of going into cells, it can cause problems:

Higher risk of Alzheimer's disease (in diabetes, hyperinsulinemia doubles your risk for AD compared to people without diabetes).

Obesity

Over time, high blood glucose levels damage your eyes, kidneys, nerves or heart.

ALL hormones work in synergy with one another. The hormone you have the most control over is insulin. This is regulated by your diet.

What Causes Insulin Resistance and Diabetes?

A Sedentary Lifestyle

Calorie restriction, skipping meals, diet pills and a crap diet of fast foods, boxed, canned or microwaved foods. Unbalanced meals, high in carbohydrates, sugar and a low intake of fats and protein.

Drinking soft drinks and fruit juices.

Elevated lypogenic (fat storing) enzymes and decreased lypolytic (fat burning) enzymes

Lack Of quality Sleep

Stress and altered hormonal levels. Years of high adrenaline and/or cortisol levels due to poor nutrition and lifestyle habits.

Diet And Nutrition For Insulin Resistance/Type Ii Diabetes:

Allowed fruits in moderation include: tomatoes, avocados, berries, grapefruit, lemons, limes

Avoid agave syrup,, HFCS, Nutra Sweet and

Aspartame products as they may trigger diabetes and obesity.

Cut carbohydrates and increase protein. Eat a diet of organic proteins, non-starchy vegetables and fats (fats slow down the insulin spike)

Eliminate all boxed, canned and microwavable foods.

Eliminate all refined carbohydrates, grains, dairy products, fast-acting sugars (fruit juices, soft drinks, high glycemic fruits and starchy vegetables), hydrogenated fats, alcohol, caffeine and tobacco).

Lemon and lime juice reduce the insulin index of the meal due to the flavonoids.

If it does not run around in the field, swim, fly or is not green - do not eat it!

Small mini meals 5-7x daily. Include smart fats and protein at each meal.

Sweeten with stevia, an herb, instead of sugar. Stevia will not elevate blood sugars.

Supplemental Nutrients For Insulin Resistance/Type II Diabetes:

- ✓ Vitamin D - Bio D Mulsion Forte
- ✓ Chromium
- ✓ R-Alpha Lipoic Acid (lowers glucose levels up to 30%)

- ✓ Omega-3 Fish oil with 400 I.U. mixed tocopherols
- ✓ Bio-Glycozyme Forte (use with hypoglycemia)
- ✓ Fiber
- ✓ GlucoBalance (use with elevated triglycerides and ' blood sugar)
- ✓ ADHS (consider with increased glucose or triglycerides, adrenal cortical hyperfuntion.

Research and clinical feed back indicates that 7 Keto-DHEA is often effective in helping to ameliorate increased glucose levels. In addition, the 7-keto DHEA will not convert androgens to estrogens.

Resveratrol

Silymarin, an antioxidant that can improve liver function (especially the insulin resistant-liver cells) and blood sugar levels, have shown great promise in the effort to fully restore insulin sensitivity.

Zinc, magnesium and potassium deficiencies lead to insulin resistance.

Improves insulin sensitivity: CoQ 10, L-Carnitine, Taurine, L-Arginine, Glutathione

Supplemental Botanicals For Insulin Resistance/Diabetes:

Fenugreek/Flax seed Potion for diabetes and insulin resistance:

- ✓ Take on an empty stomach first thing in the AM
- ✓ 1 T. freshly ground fenugreek seeds
- ✓ 1 T. freshly ground flax seeds
- ✓ 1 T. Liquid chlorophyll
- ✓ 16 ounces water

Gymnema Sylvestre before meals helps repair the pancreas and damage to liver and kidneys. Studies show that it may be able to help repair damage that has been done to the pancreas, as well as reduce the amount of insulin many diabetics need to maintain normal blood sugar levels. There is also research showing that it can reduce triglyceride levels and aid in weight loss.

- ✓ Bitter Gourd
- ✓ Banaba Tree Extract
- ✓ Grape Seed Extract
- ✓ Cinnamon - add to coffee with organic heavy cream to make you more insulin sensitive. Coffee has polyphenols which protect you from diabetes.
- ✓ Tea: Green tea, Pau d' arco, Astragalus, Burdock, Fenugreek

Lifestyle Protocol For Insulin Resistance/Type Ii Diabetes:

Ensure healthy gut flora. Consider a CDSA (comprehensive digestive stool analysis).

Get to bed by 10pm and get up no earlier than 6am. Lack of sleep disturbs lipid profile, glucose metabolism, androgen production and blood pressure, immune system and memory.

Glucose levels are influenced by carbohydrate intake, stress, glandular and liver function. Serum Glucose: Optimum range - 80-95 mg/dL. 105 and = adrenal issues

Monitor blood glucose levels at least 2 times a day and before eating meals. If you are exercising you will need to test your glucose levels more frequently.

Obtain fasting serum glucose and insulin levels.

Rule out food allergies with increased or decreased blood sugar.

Rule out heavy metal burdens, pesticides, other xenobiotics and inoculations. These can be locus to pancreatic dysfunction resulting in diabetes or hypoglycemia.

Take Care of Your Eyes - Diabetes is a leading cause of blindness. It can lead to Retinopathy and other eye problems such as cataracts.

Exercise Protocol For Insulin Resistance/Type Ii Diabetes:

Begin some form of exercise routine. Walking is

excellent for diabetes. A daily 3mph brisk walk decreases diabetes risk by 50%!

Strength training is far superior to steady state aerobic exercise to prevent obesity and improve insulin resistance. Steady state aerobic exercise 'cortisol levels which 'insulin levels.

The power of being active should never be underestimated: from a short five minute walk to forty-five minute strength training sessions, it all counts towards reducing and eliminating the pre-diabetes (insulin resistance) syndrome.

RESISTING INSULIN RESISTANCE

It seems that almost every day a new association between diet and health is discovered. Certain food groups have been shown in reliable studies to decrease the risk of various conditions; for example, the high lycopene content of tomatoes helps to prevent prostate cancer, and calcium-containing foods such as yoghurt and broccoli delay the onset of osteoporosis.

Other foods have been shown to cause, or aggravate, particular conditions. People with high blood pressure are routinely advised to cut down on salt intake. Gout sufferers are all too aware of the impact that some foods, especially drinks like beer (even alcohol-free beer!) have on their joints.

The problem with these food-health relationships, is that they are not very specific, or predictable. How many tomatoes must you eat, and for how long, for it to have a protective effect on your prostate? Assuming, of course, that you are a man and therefore would have one of these. And how much yoghurt and broccoli should you eat to help delay the onset of osteoporosis? Nobody seems to know the answers to these problems, and so it is generally recommended that we eat as much of the protective food types as we can, while avoiding the less favourable things like salt and saturated fats.

Recommendations like these seem to be a bit too vague for my liking. In this era of precise measurements and percentages, it could be expected that someone would be able to prescribe a daily or weekly portion of the particular food group required to decrease the risk of having a condition by a precise percentage. But this is just not possible. Confounding factors such as genetics need to be taken into account; if you have a family history of an illness you may have a genetic predisposition to having the condition yourself, no matter what you do. And genetics is generally too complex a subject to be able to make very accurate predictions. So any recommendations regarding eating certain foods to prevent disease should read something like this: " Eat such-and-such food, and you may be able to make a slight difference to your overall risk of developing the condition, unless your genes say otherwise, and who can tell if this is the case?" Some prediction!

However, there is one condition where lifestyle and diet will always have a predictable impact on its severity and course, and that is insulin resistance.

"What?" you say. "Never heard of it." And most people haven't heard of it, despite the fact that it is one of the most prevalent conditions in the world today. It is more common than diabetes; in fact, insulin resistance is the cause of type 2 diabetes, and has been estimated to affect about one in four people.

insulin resistance is a complex entity, which involves a spectrum of conditions ranging from excess weight around the waist, to type 2 diabetes mellitus. It is the single cause of conditions such as metabolic syndrome, polycystic ovarian syndrome and type 2 diabetes, and is strongly associated with high blood pressure, cholesterol abnormalities, gout, and most frighteningly, sudden death, especially in middle-aged women. In short, it is a medical time bomb.

Its origins are not always clear-cut either. Insulin resistance tends to run in families - although not everyone in the same family is necessarily equally affected. A brother may never show any symptoms of the illness, while his sister may have significant weight problems and go on to develop type 2 diabetes at the age of forty. Or vice versa. Why this happens is not always apparent, although diet and lifestyle do play very significant roles in the progression of the condition.

Insulin resistance may also be "acquired"; in other words it develops in an individual with no family background of insulin resistance and its associated conditions. This usually occurs in people who are overweight for whatever reasons. It has been estimated that half of all people who are significantly overweight have insulin resistance!

It may be because of this very obvious association between insulin resistance and excess weight that, despite the fact that insulin resistance is largely a genetic disorder, it is very responsive to dietary and lifestyle changes, especially those that result in significant (i.e. more than 2-5 kilograms) weight loss. Fantastic news for those who are not very fond of taking tablets!

In fact, exercise and diet were shown by the Diabetes Prevention Program to be almost twice as effective as metformin (a drug that is known to reduce insulin resistance) at reducing the risk of progressing to type 2 diabetes, which is more or less the end result of insulin resistance. And these benefits occur whether the person affected was overweight or not at the beginning of the lifestyle modification program. Strangely enough, some people with insulin resistance do not have a weight problem by ordinary standards. Instead, they may have a completely normal body mass index, and the only sign of underlying insulin resistance may be a slight thickening around the waist area.

Nevertheless, the end result of the appropriate dietary modification is the same an improvement in symptoms, and a longer, healthier life. In a world where people are becoming more interested and involved in taking control of their bodies and their health, this is excellent news. A do-it-yourself cure that really works!

Having said all this, just a word of caution. Weight loss should be approached carefully. Conventional low calorie, low fat and high carbohydrate diets do not work very well for people with insulin resistance, and crash diets work well for nobody. An appropriate diet, a bit of mild exercise, and a slow, gentle loss of weight are all that is needed to make a huge difference to your health. And to the health of those around you. Please remember that family members of people with diabetes are likely to have insulin resistance too, and need to be made aware of this possibility. With insulin resistance and diabetes, prevention is always better than cure! Dr. Guin Van Niekerk qualified as a medical doctor at the University of Cape Town in 1997. It was while working a few years later as a general practitioner that she developed a strong interest in insulin resistance and its associated conditions. She subsequently ran a small metabolic syndrome clinic for her patients and discovered that the concept of insulin resistance was largely unknown to the public.

INSULIN RESISTANCE AS IT RELATES TO WEIGHT GAIN

The relation of insulin resistance to weight gain is now well-accepted by medicine. Insulin resistance certainly promotes weight increases, particularly along the waist line. But it becomes a vicious cycle in that as we gain weight, further insulin resistance is promoted. The accepted definition of insulin resistance is the inability of some cells to take in and store glucose as fat. It happens when these cells literally don't respond to insulin as they normally should.

With insulin resistance, glucose remains in the blood stream (it can't go where it's supposed to: the cells), so to maintain balance in the blood more insulin is added to stabilize blood glucose. Besides weight gain, the other symptom will be lack of energy, as the body cannot use stored fat for energy. If the situation isn't reversed, insulin becomes less and less effective, diabetes sets in.

Genetics is believed to play a major role in a person's susceptibility to the condition, and the amount of exercise a person takes on is also important. But here we will talk about diet, and the foods that are most apt to trigger the problem. Carbohydrates have the largest impact on insulin secretion, followed by protein. People may be surprised that fats have little or no impact on insulin secretion. Although not all people respond the same to any diet, we will generalize here by describing how the following foods affect insulin resistance:

1. Carbohydrates. We know that people who experience the condition metabolize carbohydrates abnormally. This may have an effect on weight gain. In a 12 week study of obese women who all experienced insulin resistance, those that were put on a calorie-controlled reduced carbohydrate diet lost 19.6 pounds. This is about 3.5 pounds more than those only on a reduced fat diet.

Incidentally, this test was conducted with a prepared meals program, which makes the structured diets easy to control and maintain for dieters. Controlling your diet is vital for those fighting diabetic issues that result in weight gain. Fortunately one can find meal programs that are specifically designed for diabetics.

2. Proteins. There have been animal tests that insulin resistance was found in the branched-chain amino acids, but particularly so when combined with a high level of fat in the diet. The key for most people here is to not eat protein past what your energy needs require. We get branched-chain amino acids from meat, and also dairy products and legumes. They are important for muscle recovery.

3. Fats. Typically when a doctor puts a person on a weight loss program it will be a low-fat diet. But when it comes to insulin resistance, it is now commonly believed that saturated fats do not play any role in the affliction. There is some confusion when it comes to Tran's fats. There is no doubt that these fats interfere with insulin receptors and with insulin resistance. Confusion may exist when people confuse saturated fats with Tran's fats.

4. Fiber. By increasing insoluble fiber intake, a test found that after three days there was a significant improvement in insulin sensitivity. By keeping insoluble fiber consumption above 30 grams a day and decreasing carbohydrates and proteins, especially meats, will be a great way for most people to ward off diabetes

EXERCISE CAN REDUCE INSULIN RESISTANCE, HEALTH RISKS AND DEPRESSION

It's common knowledge that exercise can reduce the risk of heart disease, type 2 diabetes, hypertension, cholesterol problems, cancer, and more. Underlying those diseases is insulin resistance. Exercise reduces health risks by making skeletal muscle more sensitive to insulin, effectively reducing the resistance.

Insulin is a hormone that's produced by the pancreas and allows glucose to enter cells for metabolism. It also has several other functions.

Under certain circumstances, someone might become insulin resistant, and the cells no longer respond to insulin's cues. To get the job done, the body's first line of defense is to produce more insulin. This may work, and can continue to work until the production of insulin no longer outpaces the degree of resistance. (That's an extremely oversimplified description of the onset of type 2 diabetes.)

Along the way, the high levels of insulin are likely to cause a variety of health issues. So it's not insulin resistance per se that causes disease, but the extra insulin that's released to compensate. This is associated with Series 2 prostaglandins and inflammation.

What we typically learn about insulin resistance (IR) is

that it's a result of overweight. That's a true enough statement, but not the whole picture. For example, IR can be caused by genetic factors. Over 40 genetic mutations can result in someone's being born with insulin resistance or with a predisposition to it.

IR can also be the result of lifestyle factors. Lack of exercise is one obvious cause, along with diet. A high-fat diet can cause resistance to insulin through a specific mechanism, a high-sugar, high-carb diet through a different mechanism, and a high-fructose diet through yet another.

Insulin resistance isn't always a result of overweight/obesity. It can also be a cause. Cells differ in their sensitivity to insulin. The primary site of IR is skeletal muscle. How does insulin-resistant skeletal muscle behave? It doesn't allow glucose to enter the cell. The glucose ends up being transported to fat cells.

Another important site is the liver. How does an insulin-resistant liver behave? It doesn't respond to the feedback loop that tells it to stop releasing glucose, so glucose levels remain high. That glucose, too, can be transported to fat cells.

An interesting connection with depression exists, as well.

You may recall from 7th grade biology that amino acids are "the building blocks of protein." One of insulin's functions is to transport amino acids to skeletal muscle, where they can be used for a variety of functions. Those functions include immune support, formation of hormones and enzymes, insulin receptor site turnover, pH and fluid balances, wound healing, tissue growth and repair, blood protein formation, energy use, and more.

The most important function is the formation of specific brain chemicals from specific amino acids. One amino acid, tryptophan, is the precursor of serotonin. The brain chemical serotonin has become well known, due to the anti-depressant medications that have been on the market for years.

Insulin resistance interferes with the transport of tryptophan to the brain and can therefore contribute to depression.

To the degree that exercise can help reduce the incidence of insulin resistance, it can be said to help reduce the incidence of depression. This isn't as far-fetched as it sounds. In the research for my dissertation, participants completed tests for depression and anxiety, both before and after they had gone through the 8-week study. Consistently, the participants who were exercising regularly had lower scores for depression and anxiety.

I hope you've made exercise a regular part of your life. What I really hope is that you enjoy it. It's kinda cool to realize that what we love to do helps us reduce our risk for health problems along with our risk for mood issues.

INSULIN RESISTANCE AND EFFECTS ON HEALTH

According to many medical experts the epidemics we are experiencing with obesity, diabetes, cardiovascular disease and cancer have not occurred without reason. There are two very little talked about reasons that some researchers have found are contributing to a huge part of these health challenges.

Insulin resistance or Syndrome X

Excessive toxins in our food and drink in the form of excitotoxins (another topic later)

Most people have no clue what these two problems are - or the extent of the health damage we are reaping as a result of them!

Here is the TRUTH: If we are ever going to get control of our health we MUST understand these two problems!

Why? Because they can both be avoided and once they are - many of our health issues will resolve!

Here are some of the symptoms of insulin resistance.

See if you recognize any of them.

Fatigue

This is one of the most common symptoms, for some the fatigue follows a large carbohydrate meal - others are exhausted all day.

Brain Fogginess

Sometimes the fatigue is physical but other times it is mental. The inability to focus is most evident, but poor memory, loss of creativity, and even some learning disabilities can occur as a result of insulin resistance.

Low Blood Sugar

Some low blood sugar is normal throughout the day, especially if meals are not eaten on a regular schedule. However, prolonged hypoglycemia with

the above symptoms is not normal. Feeling agitated, jittery or moody that is quickly remedied with eating is also indicative.

Intestinal bloating. Most gas comes from excessive high sugar carbs. Insulin resistant people have gas - lots of it.

Sleepiness. Especially after a 20-30% carbohydrate meal.

Increased weight and fat storage...especially in the

abdominal area.

- ✓ Increased triglycerides.
- ✓ Increased blood pressure.
- ✓ Depression

If any of these sound familiar to you, perhaps you should investigate this information further.

First what is insulin resistance and how is it relevant to our health?

Insulin resistance is a condition where the cells of the body become resistant to the effects of insulin, that is - the normal response to the given the amount of insulin is reduced. As a result, higher levels of insulin are needed in order for insulin to have its effects. The resistance is seen with the bodies own insulin and if insulin is given through injection.

So why would our cells become resistant to something they were designed to accept? To put it very simply the pancreas has been overworked secreting insulin in an attempt to keep the high levels of glucose or sugar out of the blood because of the high glycemic (sugar) content of the food and drink many of us are consuming. You see - that is insulins job - to push blood sugar into our cells as it comes from the digestive system to be used for energy when we need it.

What we as individuals need to learn is - what kind of things that we are eating are causing this excessive amount of insulin to be released. We are told my some experts to eat high carbohydrate/low fat diets to be healthy and this is some of the worst advise we could listen to. What most people

apparently do not understand is that there are "good" carbohydrates and "bad" carbohydrates - at least as related to our insulin levels.

Scientists have even come up with something called the glycemic index (GI) to help us recognize which are "good "carbs and which are "bad". They have established a numerical system of measuring how much of a rise in circulating blood sugar a carbohydrate triggers the higher the number, the greater the blood sugar response. There are charts you can find on the internet that list the glycemic index of foods.

The goal we should all be striving for is to keep the GI number in the medium to low level because less insulin will be needed for these foods.

A glycemic index of 70 or more is high

- ✓ 56-69 is medium
- ✓ 55 or less is low

There are many reasons that we should adhere to a lower glycemic diet.

The health problems that will be averted is the biggest reason! Again, the key is to eat low glycemic because it will mean low insulin. It is the high insulin that is causing us the problems. Here is a list of some of them:

- ✓ obesity
- ✓ Type 2 diabetes
- ✓ high blood pressure
- ✓ high cholesterol
- ✓ osteoporosis
- ✓ arthritis
- ✓ heart disease
- ✓ certain cancers - notably breast and colon

How many of you knew that it was high insulin in your blood stream that was keeping you fat and contributing to the host of other problems I listed? Don't feel bad, neither did I until a few years ago, and neither do most other people today.

That is the problem. How can we fix something if we don't know what's broke? We are breaking our pancreas by eating too much high glycemic food but there is more!

The low fat garbage you are told to adhere to is just that...GARBAGE! Has anyone else noticed that since we have all the "no fat" or "low fat" stuff on the grocery shelves we are fatter than ever!

There is a very good physiologic explanation for this and further more there are many scientists who know it too!

The body's mechanisms for utilizing nutrients from food is complex and impossible for me to explain to you thoroughly (because I don't understand all of it myself) but I can share a few basic principles with you to shed some light on this insulin thing.

Insulin is secreted by the beta cells in the pancreas.

Insulins purpose is to push nutrients into the cell that are being carried around in our blood stream.

Glucose or sugar is one of those nutrients that comes from carbohydrates and is very closely monitored in the bloodstream by the body because it is needed for energy to accomplish ALL bodily activity. In fact it is the brains only food.

Glucose is toxic to the body and can cause a multitude of problems if it remains too high in the blood stream.

Extra glucose or sugar is stored as glycogen in the liver and muscle cells but in a limited amount.

Once the glycogen stores are full all extra glucose or sugar is stored in fat cells as saturated fat.

If we consume high levels of sugar (from carbohydrates) it will require high levels of insulin to move it out of the blood.

When we repeatedly have high levels of sugar requiring high levels of insulin - two things begin to happen.

- ✓ The pancreas gets tired and starts slowing down production of insulin.
- ✓ The cell membrane gets tired of letting all the insulin in and starts becoming resistant.(It should be noted that this process happens normally as we age but is greatly accelerated with high glycemic foods.)

When either or both of these things happen to a big enough degree - we have a new diabetic born.

The problem with the no fat/low fat diets is misguided because fat has no effect on insulin. In fact, the right kinds of fat play an indirect role on helping lower the insulin response to carbohydrates.

According to Barry Sears, PhD and author of A Week In the Zone, fat slows down the entry rate of carbohydrates into the bloodstream, thereby decreasing the production of insulin. Fat also sends a hormonal signal to the brain that says to "stop eating" and the fewer calories you eat - the less insulin you need. And finally fat makes food taste better! So by taking fat out of the diet (which has no effect on insulin) and replacing it with carbohydrates (which have a strong stimulatory effect on insulin), you are virtually guaranteeing that you will become fatter!

We do need to make sure that the fat we add back to the diet is mono unsaturated fat, found in such foods as olive oil, avocados, almonds, macadamia nuts and long-chain omega -3 fats found in fish and fish oils.

This seems too easy to fix! There are tons of good low and medium glycemic foods that we can fill our bellies with- especially if it means we won't be as susceptible to all those chronic diseases and we can keep insulin resistance at bay!

Reference: A Week in the Zone by Barry Sears, pHD

Karen Phelps specializes in education that helps individuals make their own informed health choices. She is knowledgable in essential oils, glyconutrients, and general nutritional practices that can optimize health

HOW INSULIN RESISTANCE AFFECTS WEIGHT LOSS

Although it is an undeniable fact that diet plays a significant role in making people becoming overweight, there are however several other factors which need to be taken into consideration due to the fact that they influence weight gain in one way or the other.

For instance, our metabolic health - the state of the different chemical reactions related to the production of energy and other products needed to sustain life from consumed food - can actually be regarded as one major weight loss factor which is not only affected by diet but equally by other factors such as stress, sleep, and exercise.

The amount and type of food that an individual eats has a significant role to play in his or her metabolism and the ability of the body to make use of that food. As a way of illustration, high glycemic index carbohydrate foods are generally known to be rapidly absorbed into the bloodstream leading to an almost instant increase in blood sugar levels. However, once the body notices an excess amount of glucose in the bloodstream, it secretes insulin from specialized cells in the pancreas to salvage the situation and in doing so maintain its metabolic health.

Closely related to the effect of diet on weight loss, this article takes a look at the concept known as insulin resistance, its causes and how it impinges on individual's ability to effectively lose weight.

Insulin's Functions

Insulin is a hormone produced by specialized cells in the pancreas and its major role is actually to regulate the metabolism of carbohydrates, fats, and proteins. Insulin is particularly known for its assistance in controlling blood glucose (sugar) levels through the removal of any excess amount of glucose from the bloodstream and the storage of it as either glycogen in liver and muscle cells or as fat in fat cells.

Putting it more succinctly, one of insulin's basic role is to transport excess blood sugar out of the bloodstream through binding with receptors on cell membranes and allowing glucose (and other nutrients) to flow into the cells for the body to use as energy. Thus insulin serves as a gatekeeper for glucose getting into body cells.

However, unhealthy eating lifestyles especially overeating caused by either "conditioned response" (a learned habit) or "emotional eating" often leads to increased blood glucose levels which make the body to secrete additional insulin as a way of attempting to maintain equilibrium in its metabolic health.

Generally, excess insulin secretion promotes excessive

storage of glucose as fat in the body. Nevertheless, this situation can over time degenerate into one where insulin receptors may become less responsive to the effect of insulin.

Development of Insulin Resistance

If there is a cycle of fluctuating elevated levels of glucose in the bloodstream (caused by excessive consumption of high glycemic index carbohydrate-containing foods) and a counteracting secretion of insulin by the pancreas, with time, this interplay can result in insulin receptors becoming "de-sensitized" or "numbed" to the effect of insulin. This condition is what is generally referred to as insulin resistance.

Insulin resistance can therefore be regarded as a situation in which normal amount of insulin secretion becomes ineffective at producing an insulin response from muscle, liver, and fat cells. The cells of the body in this condition have essentially become incapable of responding adequately to insulin to the degree they normally should.

Due to this non-responsiveness, a situation is created whereby the pancreas is forced to secrete more and more insulin in order to control and normalize blood glucose levels. The only way that the body can overcome this difficulty is for the pancreas to produce enough insulin to bring the situation under control.

Unfortunately, not everybody is capable of producing sufficient amounts of insulin, a situation which inevitably results in a constant elevated blood glucose levels leaving the person feeling tired and cranky. Insulin resistance basically changes the way in which glucose and fat are metabolized by the body and is considered to encourage the excessive storage of fat in major fat-storage areas such as the hips, thighs, and stomach.

Furthermore, insulin resistance is a precursor to Type II Diabetes which has a 90% prevalence rate among those with diabetes. It is also noteworthy to mention that nearly everyone with a fatty liver has some degree of insulin resistance, and that 90% of people with diabetes have fatty livers. Moreover, it is estimated that about 80 million Americans suffer from insulin resistance.

Besides diet, another contributor to insulin resistance may be the lack of adequate sleep. A recent Boston study of twenty healthy men, aged between 20 and 35, found that lack of adequate sleep during a one-week period was able to cause a 20% drop in insulin sensitivity. Another independent study also observed that eight out of their nine subjects showed markers of insulin resistance after just about three nights of lack of deep sleep.

In summary, it can be deduced that the more fatty tissues an individual has, the more insulin resistant the body cells may become thereby making it even more difficult for the individual to be able to effectively lose weight.

Insulin resistance in and of itself can therefore be considered a very serious problem confronting a lot of individuals trying to lose weight. However, since an individual's dietary lifestyle has been shown to have a significant influence on insulin resistance, adopting healthier eating habits in conjunction with getting more actively involved in physical exercise and having more adequate night sleep can help in restoring insulin sensitivity.

DIET FOR INSULIN RESISTANCE

Calories

When trying to lose weight to reverse insulin resistance, you must eat fewer calories than you currently consume. Use an online food diary to help you count your usual calorie intake. Decreasing your daily intake by 500 calories produces a 1-pound weekly weight loss.

Grains

Grains are an important source of energy on your diet plan. How much you need to eat each day depends on your weight loss calorie needs. For a 1,600- to 2,000-calorie diet, aim for six to eight servings a day. Eat fewer servings if you need fewer calories. A grain serving includes one slice of bread or 1/2 cup of cooked rice. Most of your grains should come from whole grains, such as whole-grain breads and cereals, to maximize nutrient and fiber intake.

Fruits And Vegetebles

Fruits and vegetables are filling and low in calories. On your insulin resistance diet plan, eat three to five servings of vegetables each day and four to five servings of fruit. A vegetable serving is equal to 1 cup of raw vegetables or 1/2-cup cooked, while a serving of fruit is equal to a medium piece of whole fruit or

1/2 cup of fresh cut fruit.

Protein

Protein choices on your DASH diet for insulin resistance include poultry, fish and lean red meat. Choosing leaner sources of protein reduces your intake of calories and saturated fat. You should limit your daily intake of protein foods to 3 to 6 ounces a day.

Dairy Foods

Dairy foods provide protein and calcium. You should get two to three servings of dairy foods a day on your insulin resistance diet plan, in which 1 cup of milk or 1 1/2 ounces of cheese equal one serving. Choose low-fat and nonfat dairy foods to limit both fat and calories.

Nuts, Seeds And Legumes

Nuts, seeds and legumes are nutrient-rich foods that provide protein, essential vitamins and fiber. On your diet plan, get three to five servings of these foods each week. One-third cup of nuts or 1/2 cup of cooked legumes is considered one serving.

Fats And Oils

Fat is a concentrated source of calories; portion size is important when watching your calorie intake. On your diet plan, get two to three servings of fat a day, which is 1 teaspoon of oil or 2 tablespoons of salad dressing.

So-called "good" fats, such as olive oil or vegetable oil, are healthier choices.

You have probably heard a lot about diabetes. Diabetes is a condition that results when insulin, a hormone, is unable to perform its tasks. The cells that produce insulin are situated in the pancreas. Insulin resistance occurs when the cells of the body are unable to follow the tasks regulated by insulin, which basically includes controlling the metabolism of carbohydrates, proteins and fats in the body. Being diagnosed with diabetes is heredity and also depends on the health of a person. For example, if he is obese, under stress or is very ill for long periods, he may face this problem. Because of this, it is essential to follow a proper diet for insulin resistance, which ensures that the blood glucose level does not increase.

Nowadays, many clinics and doctors lay special emphasis on the diet for insulin resistance. The diet basically consists of low carbohydrates, and moderate proportions of proteins and fats. People following this diet should not include white rice in their diet or artificial sweeteners. Your main source of carbohydrate should include vegetables mostly, which should be cooked lightly not using too much oil. Vegetables that can be used in the diet regularly include cucumber, cabbage, turnips, mushroom, cauliflower, radish and garlic.

When it comes to the proteins, the diet for insulin

resistance requires the patient to take small portions of fish, chicken, beef and buffalo, etc.

Fats, on the other hand, can be acquired by eating eggs but their limit should not exceed above 7 per week. Diet for insulin resistance can also include the usage of various types of nuts like cashews, walnuts and almonds.

The main idea behind the diet for insulin resistance is to ensure that large intake of carbohydrate with protein is avoided. A proper diet for insulin resistance should consist of an egg accompanied with vegetables, while at dinner, proteins can be added to the diet by consuming fish and getting carbohydrates from vegetables as mentioned previously. In the night time, you can have a stake which will add fats to your diet.

Things that should be avoided in the diet for insulin resistance include getting rid of carbohydrates like potatoes, white rice, candies, cookies, whole brown rice, tortilla and crackers. Replace these with non-starchy vegetables and fruits as mentioned above. Similarly, cut down on the salt consumption and drink lots of water. This diet will surely help in making sure that your diet and health are maintained. Diabetes can be cured, but the perfect and immaculate remedy is care.

INSULIN RESISTANCE AND EFFECTS ON HEALTH

According to many medical experts the epidemics we are experiencing with obesity, diabetes, cardiovascular disease and cancer have not occurred without reason. There are two very little talked about reasons that some researchers have found are contributing to a huge part of these health challenges.

Insulin resistance or Syndrome X

Excessive toxins in our food and drink in the form of excitotoxins (another topic later)

Most people have no clue what these two problems are - or the extent of the health damage we are reaping as a result of them!

Here is the TRUTH: If we are ever going to get control of our health we MUST understand these two problems!

Why? Because they can both be avoided and once they are - many of our health issues will resolve!

Here are some of the symptoms of insulin resistance. See if you recognize any of them.

Fatigue

This is one of the most common symptoms, for some

the fatigue follows a large carbohydrate meal - others are exhausted all day.

Brain Fogginess

Sometimes the fatigue is physical but other times it is mental. The inability to focus is most evident, but poor memory, loss of creativity, and even some learning disabilities can occur as a result of insulin resistance.

Low Blood Sugar

Some low blood sugar is normal throughout the day, especially if meals are not eaten on a regular schedule. However, prolonged hypoglycemia with

the above symptoms is not normal. Feeling agitated, jittery or moody that is quickly remedied with eating is also indicative.

Intestinal bloating. Most gas comes from excessive high sugar carbs. Insulin resistant people have gas - lots of it.

Sleepiness. Especially after a 20-30% carbohydrate meal.

Increased weight and fat storage...especially in the abdominal area.

- ✓ Increased triglycerides.
- ✓ Increased blood pressure.
- ✓ Depression

If any of these sound familiar to you, perhaps you should investigate this information further.

First what is insulin resistance and how is it relevant to our health?

Insulin resistance is a condition where the cells of the body become resistant to the effects of insulin, that is - the normal response to the given the amount of insulin is reduced. As a result, higher levels of insulin are needed in order for insulin to have its effects. The resistance is seen with the bodies own insulin and if insulin is given through injection.

So why would our cells become resistant to something they were designed to accept? To put it very simply the pancreas has been overworked secreting insulin in an attempt to keep the high levels of glucose or sugar out of the blood because of the high glycemic (sugar) content of the food and drink many of us are consuming. You see - that is insulins job - to push blood sugar into our cells as it comes from the digestive system to be used for energy when we need it.

What we as individuals need to learn is - what kind of things that we are eating are causing this excessive amount of insulin to be released. We are told my some experts to eat high carbohydrate/low fat diets to be healthy and this is some of the worst advise we could listen to. What most people apparently do not understand is that there are "good" carbohydrates and "bad" carbohydrates - at least as related to our insulin levels.

Scientists have even come up with something called the glycemic index (GI) to help us recognize which are "good "carbs and which are "bad". They have established a numerical system of measuring how much of a rise in circulating blood sugar a carbohydrate triggers the higher the number, the greater the blood sugar response. There are charts you can find on the internet that list the glycemic index of foods.

The goal we should all be striving for is to keep the GI number in the medium to low level because less insulin will be needed for these foods.

A glycemic index of 70 or more is high

- ✓ 56-69 is medium
- ✓ 55 or less is low

There are many reasons that we should adhere to a lower glycemic diet.

The health problems that will be averted is the biggest reason! Again, the key is to eat low glycemic because it will mean low insulin. It is the high insulin that is causing us the problems. Here is a list of some of them:

- ✓ obesity
- ✓ Type 2 diabetes

- ✓ high blood pressure
- ✓ high cholesterol
- ✓ osteoporosis
- ✓ arthritis
- ✓ heart disease
- ✓ certain cancers - notably breast and colon

How many of you knew that it was high insulin in your blood stream that was keeping you fat and contributing to the host of other problems I listed? Don't feel bad, neither did I until a few years ago, and neither do most other people today.

That is the problem. How can we fix something if we don't know what's broke? We are breaking our pancreas by eating too much high glycemic food but there is more!

The low fat garbage you are told to adhere to is just that...GARBAGE! Has anyone else noticed that since we have all the "no fat" or "low fat" stuff on the grocery shelves we are fatter than ever!

There is a very good physiologic explanation for this and further more there are many scientists who know it too!

The body's mechanisms for utilizing nutrients from food is complex and impossible for me to explain to you thoroughly (because I don't understand all of it myself) but I can share a few basic principles with you to shed some light on this insulin thing.

Insulin is secreted by the beta cells in the pancreas.

Insulins purpose is to push nutrients into the cell that are being carried around in our blood stream.

Glucose or sugar is one of those nutrients that comes from carbohydrates and is very closely monitored in the bloodstream by the body because it is needed for energy to accomplish ALL bodily activity. In fact it is the brains only food.

Glucose is toxic to the body and can cause a multitude of problems if it remains too high in the blood stream.

Extra glucose or sugar is stored as glycogen in the liver and muscle cells but in a limited amount.

Once the glycogen stores are full all extra glucose or sugar is stored in fat cells as saturated fat.

If we consume high levels of sugar (from carbohydrates) it will require high levels of insulin to move it out of the blood.

When we repeatedly have high levels of sugar requiring high levels of insulin - two things begin to happen.

- ✓ The pancreas gets tired and starts slowing down production of insulin.
- ✓ The cell membrane gets tired of letting all the insulin in and starts becoming resistant.(It should be noted that this process happens

normally as we age but is greatly accelerated with high glycemic foods.)

When either or both of these things happen to a big enough degree - we have a new diabetic born.

The problem with the no fat/low fat diets is misguided because fat has no effect on insulin. In fact, the right kinds of fat play an indirect role on helping lower the insulin response to carbohydrates.

According to Barry Sears, PhD and author of A Week In the Zone, fat slows down the entry rate of carbohydrates into the bloodstream, thereby decreasing the production of insulin. Fat also sends a hormonal signal to the brain that says to "stop eating" and the fewer calories you eat - the less insulin you need. And finally fat makes food taste better! So by taking fat out of the diet (which has no effect on insulin) and replacing it with carbohydrates (which have a strong stimulatory effect on insulin), you are virtually guaranteeing that you will become fatter!

We do need to make sure that the fat we add back to the diet is mono unsaturated fat, found in such foods as olive oil, avocados, almonds, macadamia nuts and long-chain omega -3 fats found in fish and fish oils.

This seems too easy to fix! There are tons of good low and medium glycemic foods that we can fill our bellies with- especially if it means we won't be as susceptible to all those chronic diseases and we can keep insulin resistance at bay!

Reference: A Week in the Zone by Barry Sears, pHD

Karen Phelps specializes in education that helps individuals make their own informed health choices. She is knowledgable in essential oils, glyconutrients, and general nutritional practices that can optimize health.

INSULIN RESISTANCE SYNDROME BASICS

Insulin resistance syndrome is basically a collection of health conditions which put you at a general heightened risk for developing diabetes and to a certain extent heart disease. Insulin resistance syndrome is also periodically referred to as syndrome X because it is a little mysterious and not really one condition but a basket of many conditions where a mix of conditions is represented.

As the name of the syndrome suggests one of the most major conditions associated with this syndrome is the body's resistance of insulin. This is where the body starts responding less and less to its own insulin production. As the body's response lessens a greater capacity of insulin production is required to metabolize glucose from the blood. If not enough insulin can be produced blood sugar levels begin to rise which is not a good thing for the body. If this begins to happen the syndrome begins feeding off of itself making things worse and worse as time passes.

Other indicators of insulin resistance syndrome or syndrome X include low HDL cholesterol levels. HDL cholesterol is sometimes known as good cholesterol because it works to clean LDL or bad cholesterol out of the blood stream. When HDL cholesterol levels are low bad cholesterol can accumulate and increase the risk for heart disease or stroke. The body's resistance of insulin can easily be treated with increases in activity levels or exercise and so too can low levels of HDL cholesterol. This is the strange irony of this disease. Treating the syndrome can effectively treat most of the underlying conditions that comprise the syndrome.

When insulin resistance syndrome is present many times high blood pressure and high levels of triglycerides are usually present as well. The very nature of syndrome X implies that that not all conditions are present but typically many are including these. If you are experiencing both poor levels of triglycerides and hypertension than this too is contributing to syndrome X.

Another hallmark of insulin resistance syndrome is low activity levels in the person as well as an above average quantity of belly fat. Despite that fact that fat can be spread across the body rather than just the belly quite often people with insulin resistance syndrome carry most of their extra weight in their bellies primarily. Increasing activity levels as well as watching what you eat both helps to decrease body weight and also aids in the reversal of syndrome X.

What is obvious in the statistics of patients who suffer from syndrome X is that they are prone to developing diabetes. In fact each component by itself plays a part in increasing those risks and as the basket of conditions increases so too does the risks for developing diabetes. Along the way many of these conditions also play a role in increasing the risks for developing heart disease and often people with insulin resistance syndrome fall victim to heart disease and strokes before diabetes ever sets is. This is why it is very important to recognize insulin resistance syndrome before major health problems arise.

As previously stated most of the conditions that make up insulin resistance syndrome are treatable with exercise and changing one's diet. Unfortunately there's not much else that can do done. There are medications which treat to some extend individual components of the syndrome but an all encompassing solution remains elusive to medicine. If you simply remove excess calories from your diet and increase your frequency of exercise you can begin the process of reversing insulin resistance syndrome.

DOES INSULIN RESISTANCE CAUSE DIABETES?

The American Medical Association Journal had a review article which stated that 25% of adults in the US are suffering from the effects of Metabolic Syndrome also known as Syndrome X or Insulin Resistance Syndrome. There is another 25% of the population who are in the process of developing insulin resistance. That adds up to 50% of the adults and 1/3 of the children are either developing or have already developed insulin resistance that will result in Metabolic Syndrome and then most of them will develop Type 2 Diabetes. That is alarming and if this trend is not reversed it will result in a catastrophic healthcare disaster. There is no way that the healthy population can pay for the cost of this healthcare disaster.

Because of a unhealthy lifestyle, including eating food that is highly process and lacking in any nutritional value, there is an epidemic of individuals developing insulin resistance. This is the metabolic sequence of events that lead to the development of this condition: due to a improper diet an individual becomes less sensitive to their own insulin (insulin insensitivity), the body begins to compensate by producing more insulin, due to the extra insulin the body is able to control the blood sugar levels at this point, as this condition progresses the body will have to continue to produce an even higher abnormal level of insulin, eventually the insulin level will begin to drop as the body is unable to keep up with the demand for more insulin, now your blood sugar level will begin to increase, next this individual will begin to develop diabetes which will develop into Type 2 Diabetes for most of the patients at this point. This individual has now developed full blown Metabolic Syndrome with all of it's devastating effects including pre-mature death if this condition is not reversed.

The 3 Main Causes of Insulin Resistance:

Poor Diet - eating food that is highly processed and lacking in any nutritional value.

Lack of activity and exercise of any aerobic value - sedentary lifestyle (couch potato).

Little or no nutritional supplements - lack of cellular nutrition from high quality vitamins and supplements.

What are the results of Insulin Resistance - Metabolic Syndrome or Syndrome X or Insulin Resistance Syndrome? Here are some of them:

- ✓ arteries begin to increase signs of premature aging - arterosclerosis,
- ✓ increase in cholesterol and triglyceride levels,
- ✓ 90% of Type 2 Diabetes caused by Insulin Resistance,

✓ Nearly all of non-genetic obesity,
✓ blood pressure increases,
✓ unable to lose and maintain body weight

Is It Possible to Reverse Insulin Resistance?

Dr. Ray Strand is my source for the information on the Triad for a Healthy Life. Actually the three parts to the Triad and they are the reverse of the same three things that caused the condition to begin with: 1. Healthy Eating, 2. Modest Aerobic Exercise 3. High Quality Supplements.

1. Healthy Eating - this is not a diet plan that you do for a short period of time, loss some weight, then slip back into your old habits and regain the weight back plus some. This is a lifestyle change, forming new habits and reaping the results of a healthier body. You will not be hunger on this eating plan even in phase 1 where you completely eliminate the high-glycemic carbohydrates and most of the good carbohydrates as you start reversing the Insulin Resistance. Some have referred to this eating style as the Mediterranean Diet. By eliminating the bad carbs you are eliminating the main cause of the problem to begin with and also breaking the cycle of what Dr. Strand calls, Carbohydrate Addiction. It is important to note that the main tool that is used to measure what a person should and should not eat is the Glycemic Index. The Glycemic Index measures the rate of how fast blood sugar or glucose levels increase after food containing carbohydrates are consumed.

If you already have Type 2 Diabetes: "If you are diabetic and on medication or insulin, you must be checking your blood sugars at least four times daily during the first few weeks of the program. If your blood sugar begins to drop and fall into the low blood sugar range (hypoglycemic range), contact your physician immediately so that he can readjust your medication." (Quote from Dr. Strand)

2. Modest Aerobic Exercise - 30 to 45 minutes, 5 times a week. Walking briskly is one of the most effective modest, low-impact aerobic exercises you can do. It is important to increase you physical activity level to add to the synergistic effect of this program or lifestyle. All three parts of this lifestyle change are important to achieve the maximum results you desire.

3. High Quality Supplements - If you are not taking a high quality vitamin and mineral supplement, you are literally starving yourself nutritionally. By in large the food we eat is lacking or totally devoid of the essential nutrients we require to maintain good health and energy. So it is critical for our wellness that we take high quality supplements.

Reversal of Insulin Resistance produces the following results:

✓ Avoiding or reversing diabetes,

✓ Ability to achieve and maintain ideal body weight,

✓ Blood sugar levels return to normal,

✓ Appetite and cravings are easier to control,

✓ No more energy highs and lows due to blood sugar spikes and lows,

✓ Blood pressure returns to normal,

✓ Mental and physical energy are easier to maintain,

✓ Energy to maintain the active lifestyle you desire,

✓ Overall health will improve - You will look good and feel good,

✓ Slowing of the aging process,

✓ Reduce or eliminate prescription drugs including insulin supplementation - only under your doctor's supervision.

✓ Cholesterol and Triglyceride levels return to normal,

Avoid the devastating effects of Diabetes including pre-mature death.

TIPS ON HOW TO TREAT INSULIN RESISTANCE

While there are so many physiological concepts that

have a lot of effect on an individual's ability to lose weight and keep it off, some however have more serious effect than others. One very important concept that should be of interest to anybody that seriously wants to lose weight is insulin resistance.

Insulin resistance can be considered to be a situation in which normal amount of insulin secretion fails to produce a corresponding effect on insulin receptors. Put another way, insulin resistance is a condition where the cells of the body (especially muscle, liver and fat cells) have become incapable of responding appropriately to insulin secretion as they should normally do.

Insulin resistance makes it very difficult for insulin to perform its normal role of removing excess glucose from the bloodstream and to store it as either glycogen in muscle and liver cells or as fat in adipose tissues (fat cells). This insensitivity of insulin receptors consequently predisposes the body to storing any excess amount of glucose as fat in fat cells due to the fact that the body keeps secreting more and more insulin in a bid to remove the excess glucose from the bloodstream.

The causes of insulin resistance have been linked mostly to unhealthy eating habits, living a sedentary lifestyle and also lack of adequate sleep; however the dietary aspect appears to be the major problem.

Fortunately, these risk factors are all well within our control and therefore insulin sensitivity can be effectively restored by making certain lifestyle changes including the ones listed hereunder.

Eating A Healthy Diet

Since excessive intake of carbohydrates have been fingered to be the major cause of insulin resistance, it therefore becomes important to keep carbohydrate consumption as low as possible. It is equally important to ensure that most of the carbohydrates come from low and moderate glycemic index types and that portion size is controlled adequately.

Exercising Regularly

A sedentary lifestyle and lack of regular physical exercise are known risk factors for developing insulin resistance and a lot of other health conditions. Regular physical activities and exercises can help the body use up more glucose and exercises in particular have been found to be helpful in the actual restoration of insulin sensitivity.

Engaging in aerobic exercises helps the body to increase the amount of oxygen available in the bloodstream and therefore the amount of body fat that can be oxidized when performing aerobic exercises during which the body normally burns fat for energy. Engaging in some form of resistance training can also help the muscles deplete their glycogen (mixture of glucose and water) stores and therefore would need to replenish it with glucose from the bloodstream.

Generally, once the level of stored body fat decreases, the body usually replaces them by removing more glucose from the bloodstream and converting them into fat for storage in fat cells as the body needs a certain amount of body fat for future energy use. Also, the dire need for the body to replenish the depleted glycogen stores of the muscles forces the insulin receptors on cell membranes to become more responsive to insulin.

Relaxing More By Reducing Stress And Sleeping Better

Chronic stress more often than not leads to sleep deprivation. Moreover, this interplay has been demonstrated to cause increase in the secretion of the stress hormone known as cortisol, which in and of itself interferes with glucose metabolism often resulting in insulin resistance.

Relaxation is one very effective stress buster that can also help improve sleeping patterns. Exercise can also help burst stress and soothe the nerves as it stimulates the body to secrete endorphins which create a "feel good" mood. You can also get this endorphin-like effect by treating yourself to a snack of good chocolate. Taking a warm bath or practicing relaxation techniques such as deep breathing can also help calm your nerves and make you sleep better.

Using Herbs And Supplements

Although there is no direct herbal remedy for insulin resistance, there are some herbal solutions that can however help to reduce blood sugar levels and in so doing reduce insulin secretion. Some good herbal recommendations includes fenugreek (reduces blood insulin and glucose levels and also lowers cholesterol); garlic (lowers blood sugar and cholesterol levels); and onion (lowers glucose levels by freeing insulin to metabolize them).

Supplements can also be beneficial in treating insulin resistance. Supplements containing essential fatty acids such as Omega-3s can help increase cell membrane fluidity and thus increase the sensitivity of insulin receptors. Of equal benefit are Vitamin D supplements; supplements that contain chromium which increases insulin effectiveness; magnesium from diet or supplements with calcium which regulate blood sugar as well as help with normal insulin functions; and also some insulin mimickers found in black tea.

Given the above considerations, insulin resistance therefore should not be something that you have to live with for the rest of your life as there are various ways through which you can overcome this condition. With the right amount of determination to change any lifestyle habit that might have been contributing to this problem, you'll be doing yourself a world of good as you'll be able to once again restore insulin sensitivity

NOT LOSING WEIGHT - COULD INSULIN RESISTANCE BE THE CAUSE?

Are you tired all the time, craving sweets /carbs, have weight around your middle that won't budge, elevated blood pressure, cholesterol, triglycerides & blood sugar? You may be fighting Insulin Resistance, a problem in your metabolism.

In a healthy metabolism, as we eat carbohydrates, insulin is secreted & takes glucose (sugar) from the carbs & carries it through the cell walls into all of our cells to use as energy/fuel. This is called an insulin pump. Our bodies then have ample energy so we feel well & have sufficient energy. The blood sugar levels are stable (no great highs or lows).

Sometimes the insulin pump is blocked at the cell wall and it cannot enter the cell. This keeps the glucose from the cells and your body doesn't have the energy it needs. This makes us feel tired. Our bodies think we need more carbs for fuel, so we get carb cravings. When we eat more sweets, more insulin is secreted but the insulin pump is only slightly able to work. The rest of the insulin & glucose floats around in our blood. We are then even more lacking in energy at the cell level and feel even more tired & lethargic. The extra insulin that is floating around triggers the body to store the extra glucose as fat. The blood sugar levels are erratic with pronounced highs & lows.

Insulin Resistance can be a never-ending cycle. The body keeps calling for more carbs to be fuel, but this makes for more insulin, less energy, and more fat deposits. This is why people feel so tired & lethargic after eating. Some people feel this as being dragged down in the afternoon of their work day. It also can lead to harmful conditions such as high blood pressure, cholesterol, triglycerides & blood sugar;

even Lupus & Chronic Fatigue.

In order to get rid of insulin resistance & its effects on the body, a lifestyle change has to happen. You can't just "try" to correct this for a while & then return to classic junk food eating... You must totally restructure your relationship with food.

Adjusting your diet is the first step to correcting this metabolic problem. A good start to stabilizing your blood sugar is to eat small moderate sized meals every 3-4 hours. A modified Low Carb diet is next. Reduce the amounts of carbohydrates you eat and focus on complex carbs like whole grains & vegetables. Also eat 3-6 oz of protein at every meal & include fruits & small amounts of fats. Cut out sugar and refined white flour as much as possible as these simple carbs break down to sugar rapidly. Be sure to drink 6-8 glasses of water a day to wash out cellular waste and help your body work better.

I have significant risks in my family history for diabetes & insulin resistance. I saw myself approaching diabetes & decided I didn't want to continue down that path. I drew a line in the sand & told myself "I have to change my lifestyle now." I was amazed that more than 90% of my sweets cravings were gone 24 hours after I had switched to this diet. I quickly began to feel less tired as well. I was able to replace sugar with sugar-free sweeteners such as Xylitol & Stevia so I didn't have to do without sweet treats.

To further control insulin resistance, supplements like vanadyl sulfate, chromium, & MCT oil can be taken to make the blood sugar levels stabilize and make the body become healthier. Adding in small amounts of exercise such as 15 minutes of brisk walking three times a week can help your body start losing that persistent weight around the middle as the insulin resistance no longer is affecting the metabolism.

COMMON FORMS OF TREATMENT FOR INSULIN RESISTANCE

Insulin resistance occurs when the body decreases its receptivity to insulin, thus diminishing insulin's beneficial effects. The condition has a number of causes and risk factors. One of the main risk factors is genetics. There are certain drugs that are risk factors as well. In fact, over the years, there have been a wide variety of factors that seem to increase the odds of a person developing insulin resistance. A partial list of these factors are - obesity, pregnancy, metabolic syndrome, stress, infection, steroid use, and some diseases.

Type II diabetes mellitus is a condition where there is intense insulin resistance. It is a condition where the body cannot properly use insulin. This is true even in the cases where the beta cells are actually producing insulin.

In a normal body, insulin will bind to receptors in the body's cells. This, in turn, induces them to use up blood glucose for energy. But, where insulin resistance is occurring, the cells either do not respond at all to insulin or they respond poorly. As a result, this causes the pancreas to produce more insulin to make the body respond.

As the cycle continues, the body produces more and

more insulin. Over time, if this scenario continues to happen without treatment, over time, insulin resistance increases, and the time will come when the pancreas ceases to produce insulin. And, when this happens, blood glucose levels will dramatically increase.

The degree of this type of insulin resistance can be diagnosed through measuring fasting insulin levels. There are also, glucose tolerance tests and the modified insulin suppression test which can help gauge the degree of the problem.

The best treatments for treating insulin resistance involves constant exercise and watching your diet. Particularly, eating more healthy foods and laying off of the junk foods that are so prevalent in the market place.

If the problem has escalated, however, dietary changes and exercise may not be enough. In this case your doctor will try a series of medications to see which ones your body will best respond to.

There are many medications used to treat insulin problems such as this. One such drug is metformin (Glucophage) which prevents the release of glucose from the liver into the blood and increases cellular sensitivity to insulin so that they remove more insulin from the blood and decrease blood sugar. Metformin has been known to halt the progress of diabetes by 31%.

Acarbose is another drug used to control the effects of insulin resistance; it slows down intestinal absorption of sugars, decreasing the need of the pancreas to produce insulin, especially after meals. Acarbose is reported to halt the progress of diabetes by 35%.

INSULIN RESISTANCE SYNDROME - WHAT ARE THE SYMPTOMS AND SIGNS?

Normally when you eat, food is absorbed into your bloodstream after it is digested and what are called beta cells in the pancreas increase putting out a hormone, called insulin, which helps remove glucose from the bloodstream so it can be used for energy. Insulin resistance means that those beta cells do not work as well as they should, so the pancreas has to pump out more insulin than normal. This can lead to high blood sugar or even Type 2 diabetes.

Insulin resistance syndrome, also called metabolic syndrome, is actually a combination of medical conditions that have been found to significantly increase the chance of someone with these conditions developing Type 2 diabetes or even heart disease and stroke.

There is no single test or medication for insulin resistance syndrome because it is not a disease per se. Rather, your doctor would look for other conditions, such as obesity, high blood sugar, high blood pressure, hardening of the arteries, and cholesterol problems to see if you may have or be likely to develop insulin resistance syndrome.

If you doctor finds a number of the conditions associated with insulin resistance syndrome, he will probably start you on a regimen to treat each condition separately in order to reduce the likelihood that those conditions, when taken together, will result in insulin resistance syndrome...which may then result in developing diabetes, heart disease and stroke.

Since a primary factor in developing insulin resistance syndrome is obesity, especially abdominal obesity, weight loss is usually the first recommended treatment, calling for both changes in diet and increased physical activity.

Multiple medications may also be required. When high blood sugar, or even Type 2 diabetes is diagnosed, patients will probably be put on medication to help the body process sugars. High cholesterol or blood pressure will also be treated to lower them.

Insulin resistance syndrome is actually preventable. A healthy lifestyle, including regular exercise and keeping your weight down through proper diet, as well as taking medications for conditions that diet and exercise have not helped enough (e.g. high blood pressure) can keep this potential deadly syndrome from developing

CAN DIABETES AND INSULIN RESISTANCE BE REVERSED?

Chances are you have been told at one point of another that diabetes is not reversible. You may have even consulted multiple physicians only to find out that the only thing you can do about your diabetes is control your blood sugar levels with medications or insulin. Chances are your doctor has told you that drugs and insulin are what will protect you from organ damage and ultimately a premature death. However, medications and insulin can actually increase your risk of a heart attack as well as increase your risk of a premature death.

The epidemic of diabetes has been accelerated by the obesity epidemic. However, what you are not being told is how you can treat it without the need for medications and insulin. There is another way to help reverse this epidemic. Type 2 diabetes, formerly known as adult onset diabetes, is a huge concern. With over 100 million people in the world and over 20 million Americans suffering from diabetes, the end of the diabetes epidemic appears to be nowhere in site. What is even more alarming is the increase of type 2 diabetes in children. Previously, type 2 diabetes was never considered a childhood illness. One in three children born today will face diabetes during their lifetime.

The scary thing is that diabetes is an entirely preventable lifestyle disease. A report in The New England Journal of Medicine, demonstrates that 91 percent of all type 2 diabetes cases can be prevented through improvements in lifestyle and diet.

The Makings Of A Diabetic Starts Early

For most people, diabetes is often undiagnosed until its later stages. Insulin resistance, which occurs when the body becomes resistant to the effects of insulin, is the primary reason many individuals will develop diabetes.

If your diet is full of empty calories, an abundance of quickly absorbed sugars and carbohydrates (such as bread, rice and pasta), the body will slowly become more and more resistant to the effects of insulin. As a result, your body will need more and more to do the same job of maintaining your blood sugar levels. If you are experiencing high insulin levels, this is the first sign that you may be heading down the road to diabetes. High insulin leads to an increased appetite. This will lead to an increase in weight gain in the abdominal region. High insulin levels serve as a warning sign, they precede type 2 diabetes by decades.

Insulin resistance and the metabolic syndrome associated with insulin resistance are often accompanied by an increase in abdominal fat, fatigue after eating, sugar cravings, high blood pressure, low HDL, high triglycerides, problems with blood clotting as well as increased inflammation throughout the body.

These are clues and symptoms that are often picked up decades before an individual is actually diagnosed with diabetes. In fact, picking up on these clues may help you to prevent diabetes entirely.

If you have a family history of diabetes, obesity, heart disease and even dementia, you are much more likely to experience problems with insulin resistance.

Early Diagnosis Is Key In Leading A Life Without Diabetes

Pre-diabetes as well as diabetes ARE reversible. Science shows that reversal of diabetes is very possible through an aggressive approach. This aggressive approach includes changes in diet, nutritional support and occasionally medications.

It is important to diagnose type 2 diabetes as early as possible. However, the reality of type 2 diabetes, is that it is often diagnosed very late. In fact, all doctors should aggressively diagnose pre-diabetes decades before a patient actually becomes a diabetic. By doing so, damage to the body can be prevented. Damage begins with even the smallest changes in insulin and blood sugar levels.

It is unfortunate that there is a continuum of risk from slightly abnormal insulin and blood sugar levels to being diagnosed an actual diabetic. This needs to be addressed as early as possible in order to prevent an individual from becoming a full blown diabetic.

One study found that anyone with a fasting blood sugar level of 87 is at increased risk of diabetes. The lowest risk group is any individual with a fasting blood sugar level of less than 81. However, most doctors are not concerned with blood sugar until it is over 110. Keep in mind that over 126 is concerned diabetic.

As a result, early testing is a must! Early testing is especially important for anyone with a family history of type 2 diabetes, central abdominal weight gain or abnormal cholesterol levels.

Do not wait until your sugar level is high; it will be too late!

Get Tested Before It's Too Late

Below is a list of tests recommended for insulin resistance as well as diabetes. These are tests that any doctor can perform and are most often covered by insurance.

- ✓ Insulin Glucose Challenge Test
- ✓ Hemoglobin A1C Test
- ✓ Lipids Profile
- ✓ NMR Lipid Profile
- ✓ High Sensitivity
- ✓ C-Reactive Protein Test
- ✓ Homocysteine Test
- ✓ Fibrinogen Test
- ✓ Ferritin Levels
- ✓ Uric Acid Test
- ✓ Liver Function Tests

5 TIPS TO HELP REVERSE INSULIN RESISTANCE AND TYPE 2 DIABETES LEADING TO LOWER BLOOD SUGAR LEVELS!

Insulin resistance is one of the greatest challenges facing many Type 2 diabetics and is the underlying problem for the majority of people with Type 2 diabetes. Diabetes and insulin are so closely connected that it is often assumed that if you have diabetes, you are not producing enough insulin. In actual fact, in Type 2 diabetes your pancreas may be producing adequate amounts of insulin, but your body refuses to let it do its job. However, the cells resist insulin's attempt to carry glucose into the muscles to be stored as energy, the glucose or sugar stays in your bloodstream. This results in elevated blood sugar levels and side effects such as headache, frequent urination, blurred vision, weak, tired feelings and irritability.

Restoring insulin sensitivity is often possible through a multi-pronged approach that takes several different factors into account.

1. Exercise: Exercise is beneficial in that it increases your muscle cells' sensitivity to insulin (as the muscles need sugar to replace energy burned during a workout and become less resistant to glucose carrying insulin). Exercise also burns fat if a sufficient level of aerobic activity is reached.

2. Diet: Diet is just as important... controlled blood sugar levels make it easier for your body to respond appropriately. A healthy diet containing protein, high fiber vegetables and whole grain carbs can help keep blood sugar levels from fluctuating, and can also assist in weight loss. Small meals throughout the day allow your body to deal with small amounts of glucose, preventing a sugar rush followed by an insulin overload, and a subsequent crash.

Eating a balanced breakfast has been shown to increase insulin sensitivity, so never skipping breakfast is a wise step to take. Stock whole grain cereal, high fiber fruit and low fat milk for a nutritious start to your day and follow up with a late morning snack.

3. Caffeine: Caffeine has been linked in some studies to insulin resistance, but coffee contains a natural countering agent. The greater danger is caffeinated diet sodas or energy drinks.

4. Adequate sleep: 7 to 8 hours of sleep each night should be standard. Individuals who suffer sleep apnea (short periods where breathing is suspended), should have their condition evaluated and treated. Don't sleep in late on weekends or your blood sugar may drop too low, causing a spike when you do eat and an insulin overreaction that could be resisted by your body. If you do want to catch a little more sleep, eat a small high protein snack before crawling back into bed.

5. De-stress: Stress releases a hormone called cortisol, which promotes lethargy, weight gain, and insulin resistance. Try to recognize and eliminate known sources of stress in your life, and adjust your attitude to deal with ones that cannot be eliminated.

Following the tips above can help you decrease your resistance to insulin and help you to lose weight resulting in lower blood sugar levels.

14 NATURAL WAYS TO IMPROVE YOUR INSULIN SENSITIVITY

Insulin is an essential hormone that controls your blood sugar levels.

It's made in your pancreas and helps move sugar from your blood into your cells for storage. When cells are insulin resistant, they can't use insulin effectively, leaving your blood sugar high.

When your pancreas senses high blood sugar, it makes more insulin to overcome the resistance and reduce your blood sugar.

Over time, this can deplete the pancreas of insulin-producing cells, which is common in type 2 diabetes. Also, prolonged high blood sugar can damage nerves and organs.

You're most at risk of insulin resistance if you have prediabetes or a family history of type 2 diabetes, as well as if you are overweight or obese.

Insulin sensitivity refers to how responsive your cells are to insulin. Improving it can help you reduce insulin resistance and the risk of many diseases, including diabetes.

Here are 14 natural, science-backed ways to boost your insulin sensitivity.

Get More Sleep

A good night's sleep is important for your health.

In contrast, a lack of sleep can be harmful and increase your risk of infections, heart disease and type 2 diabetes.

Several studies have also linked poor sleep to reduced insulin sensitivity

For example, one study in nine healthy volunteers found that getting just four hours of sleep in one night reduced insulin sensitivity and the ability to regulate blood sugar, compared to getting eight and a half hours of sleep.

Fortunately, catching up on lost sleep can reverse the effects of poor sleep on insulin resistance

A lack of sleep can harm your health and may increase

insulin resistance. Making up for lost sleep may help reverse its effects.

Exercise More

Regular exercise is one of the best ways to increase insulin sensitivity.

It helps move sugar into the muscles for storage and promotes an immediate increase in insulin sensitivity, which lasts 2–48 hours, depending on the exercise.

For example, one study found that 60 minutes of cycling on a machine at a moderate pace increased insulin sensitivity for 48 hours among healthy volunteers.

Resistance training also helps increase insulin sensitivity.

Many studies have found it increased insulin sensitivity among men and women with or without diabetes.

For example, a study of overweight men with and without diabetes found that when participants performed resistance training over a three-month period, their insulin sensitivity increased, independent of other factors like weight loss

While both aerobic and resistance training increase insulin sensitivity, combining both in your routine appears to be most effective

Aerobic and resistance training can help increase insulin sensitivity, but combining them in your workouts seems most effective.

Reduce Stress

Stress affects your body's ability to regulate blood sugar.

It encourages the body to go into "fight-or-flight" mode, which stimulates the production of stress hormones like cortisol and glucagon.

These hormones break down glycogen, a form of stored sugar, into glucose, which enters your bloodstream for your body to use as a quick source of energy.

Unfortunately, ongoing stress keeps your stress hormone levels high, stimulating nutrient breakdown and increasing blood sugar.

Stress hormones also make the body more insulin resistant. This prevents nutrients from being stored and makes them more available in the bloodstream to be used for energy.

In fact, many studies have found that high levels of stress hormones reduce insulin sensitivity.

This process may have been useful for our ancestors, who needed extra energy to perform life-sustaining activities. However, for people today who are under chronic stress, reduced insulin sensitivity can be harmful.

Activities like meditation, exercise and sleep are great ways to help increase insulin sensitivity by reducing stress.

Ongoing stress is linked to a greater risk of insulin resistance. Meditation, exercise and sleep are great ways to help reduce stress.

Lose A Few Pounds

Excess weight, especially in the belly area, reduces insulin sensitivity and increases the risk of type 2 diabetes.

Belly fat can do this in many ways, such as making hormones that promote insulin resistance in the muscles and liver.

Many studies support the link between higher amounts of belly fat and lower insulin sensitivity.

Fortunately, losing weight is an effective way to lose belly fat and increase insulin sensitivity. It may also reduce your risk of type 2 diabetes if you have prediabetes.

For example, a study at Johns Hopkins University found that people with prediabetes who lost 5–7% of their total weight over six months reduced their risk of type 2 diabetes by 54% for the next three years.

Luckily, there are many ways to lose weight through diet, exercise and lifestyle changes.

Excess weight, particularly in the belly area, reduces insulin sensitivity. Weight loss may help increase insulin sensitivity and is linked to a lower risk of diabetes.

Eat More Soluble Fiber

Fiber can be divided into two broad categories soluble and insoluble.

Insoluble fiber mostly acts as a bulking agent to help stool move through the bowels.

Meanwhile, soluble fiber is responsible for many of fiber's associated benefits, like lowering cholesterol and reducing appetite.

Several studies have found a link between high soluble fiber intake and increased insulin sensitivity.

For example, a study in 264 women found that those who ate more soluble fiber had significantly lower levels of insulin resistance.

Soluble fiber also helps feed the friendly bacteria in your gut, which have been linked to increased insulin sensitivity.

Foods that are rich in soluble fiber include legumes, oatmeal, flaxseeds, vegetables like Brussels sprouts and fruits like oranges.

Eating soluble fiber has many health benefits and has been linked to increased insulin sensitivity. It also helps feed the friendly bacteria in your gut.

Add More Colorful Fruit And Vegetables To Your Diet

Not only are fruits and vegetables nutritious, they also provide powerful health-boosting effects.

In particular, colorful fruits and vegetables are rich in plant compounds that have antioxidant properties

Antioxidants bind to and neutralize molecules called free radicals, which can cause harmful inflammation throughout the body.

Many studies have found that eating a diet rich in plant compounds is linked to higher insulin sensitivity.

When you're including fruit in your diet, stick to normal portion sizes and limit your intake to two pieces or less per sitting and 2–5 servings per day.

Colorful fruits and vegetables are rich in plant compounds that help increase insulin sensitivity. But be careful not to eat too much fruit in a single sitting, as some types are high in sugar.

Add Herbs And Spices To Your Cooking

Herbs and spices were used for their medicinal properties long before they were introduced into cooking.

However, it wasn't until the past few decades that scientists began examining their health-promoting properties.

Herbs and spices including fenugreek, turmeric, ginger and garlic have shown promising results for increasing insulin sensitivity.

Fenugreek seeds: They're high in soluble fiber, which helps make insulin more effective. Eating them whole, as an extract or even baked into bread may help increase blood sugar control and insulin sensitivity.

Turmeric: Contains an active component called curcumin, which has strong antioxidant and anti-inflammatory properties. It seems to increase insulin sensitivity by reducing free fatty acids and sugar in the blood.

Ginger: This popular spice is linked to increased insulin sensitivity. Studies have found that its active component gingerol makes sugar receptors on muscle cells more available, increasing sugar uptake.

Garlic: In animal studies, garlic has appeared to improve insulin secretion and have antioxidant properties that increase insulin sensitivity.

These findings for herbs and spices are promising. However, most research in this area is recent and was conducted in animals. Human studies are needed to investigate whether herbs and spices do indeed increase insulin sensitivity.

Garlic, fenugreek, turmeric and ginger may help increase insulin sensitivity. The research behind them is recent, so more studies are needed before strong conclusions can be made.

Add A Pinch Of Cinnamon

Cinnamon is a tasty spice that's packed with plant compounds.

It's also known for its ability to reduce blood sugar and increase insulin sensitivity.

For example, one meta-analysis found consuming 1/2–3 teaspoons (1–6 grams) of cinnamon daily significantly reduced both short and long-term blood sugar levels

Studies suggest that cinnamon increases insulin sensitivity by helping receptors for glucose on muscle cells become more available and efficient at transporting sugar into the cells.

Interestingly, some studies have found that cinnamon contains compounds that can mimic insulin and act directly on cells.

Cinnamon could help increase insulin sensitivity by increasing glucose transport into cells and may even mimic insulin to increase sugar uptake from the bloodstream.

Drink More Green Tea

Green tea is an excellent beverage for your health.

It's also a great choice for people with type 2 diabetes or those who are at risk of it. Several studies have found that drinking green tea can increase insulin sensitivity and reduce blood sugar

For example, an analysis of 17 studies investigated the effects of green tea on blood sugar and insulin sensitivity.

It found that drinking green tea significantly reduced fasting blood sugar and increased insulin sensitivity.

These beneficial effects of green tea could be due to its powerful antioxidant epigallocatechin gallate (EGCG), which many studies have found to increase insulin sensitivity

Drinking more green tea could help increase your

insulin sensitivity and overall health. The increase in insulin sensitivity associated with green tea could be due to the antioxidant epigallocatechin gallate.

Try Apple Cider Vinegar

Vinegar is a versatile liquid. You can clean with it or use it as an ingredient in foods, in addition to many other uses.

It's also a key ingredient in apple cider vinegar, an extremely popular beverage in the natural health community.

Vinegar could help increase insulin sensitivity by reducing blood sugar and improving the effectiveness of insulin

It also appears to delay the stomach from releasing food into the intestines, giving the body more time to absorb sugar into the bloodstream

One study found that consuming apple cider vinegar increased insulin sensitivity by 34% during a high-carb meal in people who were insulin resistant and by 19% in people with type 2 diabetes (68).

Vinegar could help increase insulin sensitivity by improving insulin's effectiveness and delaying food release from the stomach to give insulin more time to act.

Cut Down On Carbs

Carbs are the main stimulus that causes insulin blood levels to rise.

When the body digests carbs into sugar and releases it into the blood, the pancreas releases insulin to transport the sugar from the blood into the cells.

Reducing your carb intake could help increase insulin sensitivity. That's because high-carb diets tend to lead to spikes in blood sugar, which put more pressure on the pancreas to remove sugar from the blood.

Spreading your carb intake evenly throughout the day is another way to increase insulin sensitivity.

Eating smaller portions of carbs regularly throughout the day provides the body with less sugar at each meal, making insulin's job easier. This is also supported with research showing that eating regularly benefits insulin sensitivity.

The type of carbs you choose is also important.

Low-glycemic index (GI) carbs are best, since they slow the release of sugar into the blood, giving insulin more time to work efficiently

Carb sources that are low-GI include sweet potatoes, brown rice, quinoa and some varieties of oatmeal.

Eating fewer carbs, spreading your carb intake

throughout the day and choosing lower-GI carbs are smart ways to increase insulin sensitivity.

Avoid Trans Fats

If there's anything worth removing from your diet completely, it's artificial trans fats.

Unlike other fats, they provide no health benefits and increase the risk of many diseases.

Evidence on the effects of high trans fat intake on insulin resistance appears to be mixed. Some human studies have found it harmful, while others haven't.

However, animal studies have provided strong evidence linking high trans fat intake to poor blood sugar control and insulin resistance.

Because the findings are mixed for human studies, scientists can't clearly say that eating artificial trans fats increases insulin resistance. However, they are a risk factor for many other diseases, including diabetes, so they are worth avoiding.

Foods that typically contain artificial trans fats include pies, doughnuts and fried fast foods. Artificial trans fats are typically found in more processed foods.

Fortunately, in 2015 the US Food and Drug Administration (FDA) declared trans fats unsafe to eat. It gave food manufacturers three years to either gradually remove trans fats from their food products or apply for special approval.

The link between artificial trans fats and insulin resistance is stronger in animal studies than human studies. Nevertheless, it's best to avoid them since they increase the risk of many other diseases.

Reduce Your Intake Of Added Sugars

There's a big difference between added sugars and natural sugars.

Natural sugars are found in sources like plants and vegetables, both of which provide lots of other nutrients.

Conversely, added sugars are found in more highly processed foods. The two main types of sugar added during the production process are high-fructose corn syrup and table sugar, also known as sucrose.

Both contain approximately 50% fructose.

Many studies have found that higher intakes of fructose can increase insulin resistance among people with diabetes.

The effects of fructose on insulin resistance also appear to affect people who don't have diabetes, as reported in an analysis of 29 studies including a total of 1,005 normal and overweight or obese participants.

The findings showed that consuming a lot of fructose

over less than 60 days increased liver insulin resistance, independent of total calorie intake

Foods that contain lots of added sugar are also high in fructose. This includes candy, sugar-sweetened beverages, cakes, cookies and pastries.

High intakes of fructose are linked to a higher risk of insulin resistance. Foods that contain high amounts of added sugar are also high in fructose.

The idea of taking natural supplements to increase your insulin sensitivity is fairly new.

Many different supplements may increase insulin sensitivity, but chromium, berberine, magnesium and resveratrol are backed by the most consistent evidence.

Chromium: A mineral involved in carb and fat metabolism. Studies have found that taking chromium picolinate supplements in doses of 200–1,000 mcg could improve the ability of insulin receptors to reduce blood sugar.

Magnesium: A mineral that works with insulin receptors to store blood sugar. Studies have found that low blood magnesium is linked to insulin resistance. Taking magnesium may help increase insulin sensitivity.

Berberine: A plant molecule extracted from a variety of herbs including the plant Berberis. Its effects on insulin are not exactly known, but some studies have found it increases insulin sensitivity and lowers blood sugar.

Resveratrol: A polyphenol found in the skin of red grapes and other berries. It may increase insulin sensitivity, especially in those with type 2 diabetes, but its function is poorly understood

As with all supplements, there is a risk they may interact with your current medication. If you are ever unsure, it's best to check with your doctor before you start taking them.

Losing weight to improve insulin resistance

Research has found that a weight loss of 5–7 percent is enough to reduce the risk of diabetes by 58 percent in a person who has a high risk of the condition. For someone who weighs 200 pounds (lb), this would be a loss of 10–14 lb.

For a person with diabetes or a high risk of diabetes, losing weight and maintaining a healthy weight can help reduce the risk of insulin resistance, prediabetes, diabetes, and the health complications that can result.

Weight-loss tips

People with insulin resistance, prediabetes, or a high risk of diabetes need a long-term dietary and lifestyle strategy to protect their health. A "crash diet" will not reduce insulin resistance.

The CDC's National Diabetes Prevention Program emphasizes eating more healthful foods and doing at least 150 minutes of physical activity each week.

These strategies can help a person lose weight and build healthful habits for life.

Choosing healthful foods that include plenty of fresh fruits and vegetables, being mindful of portion sizes, and moderating carbohydrate intake are three of the most important factors in a sustainable, healthful diet.

The DASH eating plan, which the National Institutes of Health (NIH) developed, is a healthful, long-term diet. DASH stands for Dietary Approaches to Stop Hypertension.

The diet does not focus on calorie control but instead encourages people to eat:

- ✓ plenty of fruit and vegetables
- ✓ low-fat dairy products
- ✓ nuts and seeds
- ✓ beans and pulses

It advises people to avoid empty carbohydrates and sugars and to increase their intake of nutrient-rich foods and heart-healthy proteins.

The DASH diet is more suitable for long-term application than a crash diet or many calorie-controlled diets. This dietary approach also provides high fiber intake, which helps manage blood sugar levels by slowing the absorption of carbohydrates and reducing the need for insulin.

Other tips for reversing insulin resistance

Weight loss and a healthful diet are important ways of reducing the chance of developing insulin resistance, but adding other strategies will lower the risk further.

Quitting Smoking

Some studies have suggested that regular use of tobacco products may increase the risk of diabetes and insulin resistance. Others, however, have not found evidence of a direct link.

A 2016 study looking at the data of nearly 6,000 people concluded that there may not be a direct link between smoking and insulin resistance but that it may still play a role in causing diabetes in combination with other factors.

However, smoking is a risk factor for heart disease, lung infections, and other health conditions that are also complications of diabetes. Smoking can worsen these issues too.

For this reason, a person with insulin resistance or a high risk of diabetes should quit smoking if necessary and avoid secondhand smoke where possible. A doctor can help a person find resources and strategies to make quitting easier.

Physical Activity

Regular activity can improve insulin resistance because the muscles use up glucose from the bloodstream and do not require insulin.

The Physical Activity Guidelines for Americans recommend that adults do a minimum of 150 minutes of moderate-intensity aerobic exercise or 75 minutes of vigorous-intensity aerobic exercise each week.

For the best results, people should combine cardiovascular training with muscle-building exercises and stretching.

It is best to talk to a doctor before beginning a new exercise plan, especially if a person has not been physically active for some time.

Vitamin D

A vitamin D deficiency is common with type 2 diabetes.

Some research has found that people with diabetes are more likely to have low vitamin D levels.

However, there is not yet any evidence that taking vitamin D supplements can prevent diabetes or prediabetes. In one study, researchers have found that taking vitamin D supplements did not affect blood sugar levels in people with well-managed diabetes.

The Office of Dietary Supplements recommend that people aged 1–70 years should consume 600 international units (IU) of vitamin D a day from dietary sources.

While sunlight is by far the most concentrated source of vitamin D, dietary sources include:

- ✓ oily fish
- ✓ fortified milk and other dairy products
- ✓ fortified cereal
- ✓ egg yolks

People should ask their doctor about whether vitamin D supplementation is appropriate for them.

Sleep

Insufficient or poor-quality sleep can increase a person's risk of developing insulin resistance and type 2 diabetes.

The authors of a 2015 study noted that for people with diabetes, sleep is "an additional lifestyle behavior, important for metabolic health and energy homeostasis."

Getting plenty of sleep each day can help regulate the hormones that play a role in hunger and reduce the risk of glucose metabolism dysfunction.

Medication

Some people need medication to help improve insulin sensitivity, especially when dietary and lifestyle changes have not been effective. Doctors often prescribe metformin or other medicines for this purpose.

Takeaway

A diagnosis of insulin resistance does not automatically mean that a person has diabetes, but, without intervention, diabetes can develop.

Achieving and maintaining a suitable target weight can reduce the risk of developing type 2 diabetes.

People with insulin resistance, prediabetes, or diabetes should ask their doctor about a suitable weight-loss plan.

Healthful eating habits are crucial for losing weight, maintaining a healthy weight, and preventing insulin resistance.

DOES THE INSULIN RESISTANCE DIET ALSO HELP WEIGHT WATCHERS?

Human lifestyle has evolved from being happy and easy going to extremely nerve-racking. This has its effects on the health and well being of every individual all over the world. The illnesses which were only known to hit people in their old age are now common through the ages. The rate of high blood pressure and diabetes among youngsters is increasing alarmingly. The main reason for all these problems is hectic lifestyle and bad food habits. In such a situation the insulin resistance diet comes as a life saver.

The main purpose of insulin in the human body is to supply glucose cells to all parts of the body, thus helping to reduce the sugar from the bloodstream. Insulin syndrome is a disorder where it fails to do the expected function properly. This leads to increased blood sugar levels and may cause fatal consequences if not dealt right. Hence the insulin resistance diet plays a vital role in regulating the blood sugar levels and a sudden increase is avoided.

The insulin resistance diet comprises of low carbohydrates, moderate fat and moderate protein which is planned to slow down the digestion process and keep a check on the sugar levels. This is a very effective and natural means for people suffering from diabetes and is simple to follow. This concept is based on what our ancestors evolved eating million years ago and has the highest potential of supporting healing and preventing diseases. This diet as such facilitates a balanced food intake and can also be very beneficial for people eager to lose those extra kilos. It may take 2-3 months to establish normal insulin sensitivity but the affectivity may vary from person to person. Being obese can delay the process to reach stability in the levels.

People following the insulin resistance diet should know that this is a naturally alkalizing unlike the normal acidifying diet consumed by the masses. Once this diet is followed properly the person does not feel hungry till it is time for his/her next scheduled meal. The main foods that are

problematic and need to be avoided are starchy and refined carbohydrates. These are found in food like potatoes, simple sweets and sugars, white breads and pastas, whole grain products like tortillas, cornbreads, crackers, rice etc. All carbohydrates are not bad, but they need to be consumed along with sufficient protein during meals. Fruits can be eaten in moderation but dried fruits need to be avoided.

Food that is high in protein too has to be chosen as per an individual's metabolism. There are many who are allergic to dairy and poultry products.

Lean meats and wild fish are best options as they are

high in Omega-3 which stimulate blood flow and is very beneficial in prevention of life threatening diseases like strokes, heart attacks, arthritis and high blood pressure problems. Consumption of nuts like walnuts and almonds is healthy. The insulin resistance diet does not agree with a low fat diet and hence advises consumption of healthy oils like olive, canola, coconut and palm. Flax oil too is very good and high in Omega-3. Following basics like drinking plenty of water goes without saying.

This insulin resistance diet is becoming a hot favorite among people wanting to lose weight as it does not restrict fat and carbohydrate intake completely unlike other weight loss diets. This makes it simple to follow and does not leave the person craving for food. This diet when pursued with strong determination and a good exercise regimen will produce the desired results. People suffering from diabetes however should continue to monitor the lab values regularly to check the signs, values and symptoms of any problems.

3 REASONS THE INSULIN RESISTANT DIET DOES NOT WORK

There are 3 basic scientific reasons why the insulin resistant diet does not give you a normal blood sugar level. This diet is not based on any real scientific evidence for diabetics.

1. The first reason that this diet did not help many is that it was based on a complicated system of trying to link foods together. Normal people do not eat this way. Looking for ways to link foods lead many to not being able to find the combination so they could enjoy a meal. Also with this diet, you were given the foods you had to combine which is also not natural. Trying to find links caused many to stop the diet.

2. The diet use protein as a basis of the whole diet. Basically you can eat protein with every meal and this in some way will help lead to a balanced diet. This again is not based on any real scientific research at all. Actually this may even be very dangerous advice to a diabetic due to the fact there is a poison in the bloodstream of the diabetic. This poison is in the form of glucose. It is a spreading pollution that ruins the body and stops the circulation. This is deadly and dangerous. Many diabetic will have to have their legs cut off or will lose their eyesight. This is a very real and serious poison in the bloodstream that must be corrected quickly. The kidneys of the diabetic is weak,

this is due to the overwork trying to remove glucose by constant urinating. The insulin resistant diet works the kidneys even more since it is based on abundant protein.

3. This diet blames fat for everything and tells people to remove fat. This is bad science and very unhealthy. Research shows that the cells of a diabetic needs health fat to balance and correct the damage from the blood sugar. The truth is that most diabetes diets are based on removing sugar and fat and this is bad science that does not work. The good news is that there is a type 2 diabetes diet by a filmmaker that has been stopping diabetes. It is based on a healing of the insulin problem while people eat what they like. If you have this illness be careful of the danger of the insulin resistant diet.

14 WAYS TO LOWER YOUR INSULIN LEVELS

Insulin is an extremely important hormone that's

produced by your pancreas.

It has many functions, such as allowing your cells to take in sugar from your blood for energy.

However, too much insulin can lead to serious health problems.

Having high levels, also known as hyperinsulinemia, has been linked to obesity, heart disease and cancer.

High blood insulin levels also cause your cells to become resistant to the hormone's effects.

When you become insulin resistant, your pancreas produces even more insulin, creating a vicious cycle.

Here are 14 things you can do to lower your insulin levels.

Follow A Low-Carb Diet

Of the three macronutrients carbs, protein and fat carbs raise blood sugar and insulin levels the most.

For this and other reasons, low-carb diets can be very effective for losing weight and controlling diabetes.

Many studies have confirmed their ability to lower insulin levels and increase insulin sensitivity, compared to other diets.

People with health conditions characterized by insulin resistance, such as metabolic syndrome and polycystic ovary syndrome (PCOS), may experience a dramatic lowering of insulin with carb restriction.

In one study, individuals with metabolic syndrome were randomized to receive either a low-fat or low-carb diet containing 1,500 calories.

Insulin levels dropped by an average of 50% in the low-carb group, compared to 19% in the low-fat group.

In another study, when women with PCOS ate a lower-carb diet containing enough calories to maintain their weight, they experienced greater reductions in insulin levels than when they ate a higher-carb diet

Low-carb diets have been shown to increase insulin sensitivity and reduce insulin levels in people with obesity, diabetes, metabolic syndrome and PCOS.

Take Apple Cider Vinegar

Apple cider vinegar has been credited with preventing insulin and blood sugar spikes after eating.

This has been shown to mainly occur when vinegar is taken with high-carb foods.

A small study found that people who took about 2 tablespoons (28 ml) of vinegar with a high-carb meal experienced lower insulin levels and greater feelings of fullness 30 minutes after the meal.

Researchers believed this effect was partly due to

vinegar's ability to delay stomach emptying, leading to a more gradual absorption of sugar into the bloodstream (15Trusted Source).

Vinegar may help prevent high insulin levels after you consume meals or foods high in carbs.

Watch Portion Sizes

Although the pancreas releases different amounts of insulin depending on the type of food you eat, eating too much of any food at one time can lead to hyperinsulinemia.

This is especially a concern in obese people with insulin resistance.

In one study, insulin-resistant obese people who consumed a 1,300-calorie meal had twice the increase in insulin as lean people who consumed the same meal.

They also experienced nearly twice the increase in insulin as obese people who were considered "metabolically healthy".

Consuming fewer calories has consistently been shown to increase insulin sensitivity and decrease insulin levels in overweight and obese individuals, regardless of the type of diet they consume.

One study looked at different weight loss methods in 157 people with metabolic syndrome.

The researchers found that fasting insulin levels decreased by 16% in the group that practiced calorie restriction and 12% in the group that practiced portion control

Reducing calorie intake by portion control or counting calories can lead to lower insulin levels in overweight and obese people with type 2 diabetes or metabolic syndrome.

Avoid All Forms Of Sugar

Sugar may very well be the most important food to stay away from if you're trying to lower your insulin levels.

In one study where people overate either candy or peanuts, the candy group experienced a 31% increase in fasting insulin levels, compared to a 12% increase in the peanut group.

In another study, when people consumed jams containing high amounts of sugar, their insulin levels rose significantly more than after consuming low-sugar jams.

Fructose is found in table sugar, honey, high-fructose corn syrup, agave and syrup. Consuming large quantities of it promotes insulin resistance, which ultimately drives insulin levels higher.

One study found that people had similar insulin responses after consuming 50 grams of table sugar, honey or high-fructose corn syrup every day for 14 days.

In another study, overweight people who added high-sugar foods to their usual diet experienced a 22% increase in fasting insulin levels.

In contrast, the group who added artificially sweetened foods to their usual diet experienced a 3% decrease in fasting insulin levels

A high intake of sugar in any form has been shown to increase insulin levels and promote insulin resistance.

Exercise Regularly

Engaging in regular physical activity can have powerful insulin-lowering effects.

Aerobic exercise appears to be very effective at increasing insulin sensitivity in people who are obese or have type 2 diabetes.

One study compared two groups. One performed sustained aerobic exercise, and the other performed high-intensity interval training.

The study found that although both groups experienced improvements in fitness, only the group that performed sustained aerobic activity experienced significantly lower insulin levels.

There's also research showing that resistance training

can help decrease insulin levels in older and sedentary adults.

Combining aerobic and resistance exercise seems to be the most effective and has been shown to most greatly affect insulin sensitivity and levels.

In a study of 101 breast cancer survivors, those who engaged in a combination of strength-training and endurance exercise for 16 weeks experienced a 27% reduction in insulin levels.

Aerobic exercise, strength training or a combination of both may help increase insulin sensitivity and lower your levels.

Add Cinnamon to Foods and Beverages

Cinnamon is a delicious spice loaded with health-promoting antioxidants.

Studies in healthy people and those with insulin resistance suggest that taking cinnamon may enhance insulin sensitivity and decrease insulin levels.

In one study, healthy people who consumed about 1.5 teaspoons of cinnamon in rice pudding had significantly lower insulin responses than when they ate rice pudding without cinnamon

In another small study, young men who consumed a high-sugar drink after taking cinnamon for 14 days experienced lower insulin levels than when they consumed the drink after taking a placebo for 14 days.

It's important to note that not all studies have found that cinnamon lowers your levels or increases insulin sensitivity. Cinnamon's effects may vary from person to person.

However, including up to one teaspoon (2 grams) per day may provide other health benefits, even if it doesn't reduce your levels significantly.

Some studies have found that adding cinnamon to foods or beverages lowers insulin levels and increases insulin sensitivity.

Stay Away From Refined Carbs

Refined carbs are a major part of many people's diets.

However, research in animals and humans has found that consuming them regularly can lead to several health problems.

These include high insulin levels and weight gain.

Furthermore, refined carbs have a high glycemic index.

The glycemic index (GI) is a scale that measures a specific food's capacity to raise blood sugar. Glycemic load takes into account a food's glycemic index, as well as the amount of digestible carbs contained in a serving.

Several studies have compared foods with different glycemic loads to see if they affected insulin levels differently.

They found that eating a high-glycemic load food raises your levels more than eating the same portion of a low-glycemic load food, even if the carb contents of the two foods are similar.

In one study, overweight people followed one of two unrestricted-calorie diets for 10 weeks. After a test meal, the high-GI group had higher insulin levels than the low-GI group.

Replacing refined carbs, which are digested and absorbed quickly, with slower-digesting whole foods may help lower insulin levels.

Avoid Sedentary Behavior

In order to reduce insulin levels, it's important to live an active lifestyle.

One study of over 1,600 people found that those who were the most sedentary were nearly twice as likely to have metabolic syndrome as those who performed moderate activity at least 150 minutes per week.

Other studies have shown that getting up and walking around, rather than sitting for prolonged periods, can help keep insulin levels from spiking after a meal

A 12-week study in middle-aged sedentary women

found that the women who walked for 20 minutes after a large meal had increased insulin sensitivity, compared with women who didn't walk after a meal.

In addition, the walking group became more fit and lost body fat.

Another study looked at 113 overweight men at risk of type 2 diabetes.

The group who took the most steps per day had the greatest reduction in insulin levels and lost the most belly fat, compared to the group who took the lowest number of steps daily.

Avoiding prolonged sitting and increasing the amount of time you spend walking or doing other moderate activities can reduce insulin levels.

Try Intermittent Fasting

Intermittent fasting has become very popular for weight loss.

Research suggests it may help reduce insulin levels as effectively as daily calorie restriction.

One study found that obese women lost weight and had other health improvements following calorie-restricted intermittent fasting with either liquid or solid meals.

However, only the liquid diet significantly reduced

fasting insulin levels.

Alternate-day fasting involves fasting or dramatically reducing calories one day and eating normally the following day. Some studies have found it effectively lowers insulin levels.

In one study, 26 people who fasted every other day for 22 days experienced an impressive 57% decrease in fasting insulin levels, on average.

Although many people find intermittent fasting beneficial and enjoyable, it doesn't work for everyone and may cause problems in some people.

Intermittent fasting may help reduce insulin levels. However, study results are mixed, and this way of eating may not suit everyone.

Increase Soluble Fiber Intake

Soluble fiber provides a number of health benefits, including helping with weight loss and reducing blood sugar levels.

It absorbs water and forms a gel, which slows down the movement of food through the digestive tract. This promotes feelings of fullness and keeps blood sugar and insulin from rising too quickly after a meal.

One observational study found women who ate the highest amount of soluble fiber were half as likely to be insulin resistant as women who ate the least amount of soluble fiber .

Soluble fiber also helps feed the friendly bacteria that live in your colon, which may improve gut health and reduce insulin resistance.

In a six-week controlled study of obese older women, those who took flaxseed experienced greater increases in insulin sensitivity and lower insulin levels than women who took a probiotic or placebo.

Overall, fiber from whole foods appears to be more effective at reducing insulin than fiber in supplement form, although results are mixed.

One study found that a combination of whole food and supplemental fiber lowered insulin levels the most. Meanwhile, another found that insulin decreased when people consumed black beans but not when they took a fiber supplement.

Soluble fiber, especially from whole foods, has been shown to increase insulin sensitivity and lower insulin levels, particularly in people with obesity or type 2 diabetes.

Lose Belly Fat

Belly fat, also known as visceral or abdominal fat, is linked to many health problems.

Carrying too much fat around your abdomen promotes

inflammation and insulin resistance, which drives hyperinsulinemia.

Studies have shown that decreasing belly fat leads to increased insulin sensitivity and lower insulin levels.

Interestingly, one study found that people who lost abdominal fat retained the benefits for insulin sensitivity, even after regaining a portion of the belly fat back

Unfortunately, people with high insulin levels often find it very difficult to lose weight. In one study, those with the highest levels not only lost weight less rapidly but also regained the most weight later on (76Trusted Source).

However, there are several things you can do to lose belly fat effectively, which should help lower your insulin levels.

Losing belly fat can increase insulin sensitivity and help reduce your insulin levels.

Drink Green Tea

Green tea is an incredibly healthy beverage.

It contains high amounts of an antioxidant known as epigallocatechin gallate (EGCG).

Several studies suggest it may help fight insulin resistance.

In one study, people with high insulin levels who took green tea extract experienced a small decrease in insulin over 12 months, while those who took a placebo had an increase.

In a detailed analysis of 17 studies, researchers reported that green tea was found to significantly lower fasting insulin levels in studies considered the highest quality.

However, not all high-quality studies have shown that green tea reduces insulin levels or increases insulin sensitivity.

Several studies have found that green tea may increase insulin sensitivity and decrease insulin levels.

Eat Fatty Fish

There are many reasons to consume fatty fish like salmon, sardines, mackerel, herring and anchovies.

They provide high-quality protein, and are by far the best sources of long-chain omega-3 fats, which have all sorts of benefits.

Studies have shown they may also help reduce insulin resistance in people with obesity, gestational diabetes and PCOS.

One study in women with PCOS found a significant 8.4% decrease in insulin levels in a group who took fish oil, compared to a group who took placebo.

Another study in obese children and adolescents showed that taking fish oil supplements significantly reduced insulin resistance and triglyceride levels.

The long-chain omega-3 fatty acids found in fatty fish may help reduce insulin resistance and insulin levels.

Get the Right Amount and Type of Protein

Consuming adequate protein at meals can be beneficial for controlling your weight and insulin levels.

In one study, overweight older women had lower insulin levels after consuming a high-protein breakfast compared to a low-protein breakfast. They also felt fuller and ate fewer calories at lunch.

However, protein does stimulate insulin production so that your muscles can take up amino acids. Therefore, eating very high amounts will lead to higher insulin levels.

In addition, some types of protein appear to cause greater insulin responses than others. One study found that whey and casein protein in dairy products raised insulin levels even higher than bread in healthy people.

However, the insulin response to dairy proteins may be somewhat individual.

One recent study found that insulin levels increased similarly in obese men and women after meals containing beef or dairy.

Another study in obese adults showed a high-dairy diet led to higher fasting insulin levels than a high-beef diet.

Avoiding excessive amounts of protein, especially dairy protein, can help prevent insulin levels from rising too high after meals.

High insulin levels can lead to many health problems.

Taking steps to increase your insulin sensitivity and decrease your insulin levels may help you lose weight, lower your risk of disease and increase your quality of life.

INSULIN RESISTANCE: THE REAL REASON WHY YOU AREN'T LOSING WEIGHT

Weight problems aren't just about overeating or under exercising they're about metabolic changes that are collectively known as insulin resistance.

Many people have weight loss as one of their key resolutions. Sadly, 35 percent of people also give up on that goal before the month even ends. It's not necessarily lack of time or willpower that causes you to struggle with weight loss year after year. The real reason that you may have struggled to lose weight is insulin resistance, or a condition I call metabolism dysfunction.

So you may be thinking, "Why is it so hard for me to lose weight?" I'm doing "everything right," and yet still weight loss is difficult. Perhaps (like many of my patients) you're already following a strict diet and working out several times a week, but to no avail. The weight still won't come off -- or, worse, you are gaining weight for seemingly no reason at all! You have become resigned to being overweight.

Weight problems aren't a permanent and immovable fixture for the rest of your life. If you're finding that weight is easy to gain and hard to lose, it's not your fault! Weight problems aren't just about overeating or under exercising -- they're about metabolic changes (The MD Factor Diet, 2015) that are collectively known as insulin resistance. Lab tests conducted in my practice have confirmed that over 89 percent of my patients have this real and often undiagnosed issue. So the good news is that the right combination of diet, exercise, and will to succeed you can reverse your MD factor and finally find success in losing weight and keeping it off for good.

In a nutshell, insulin resistance is the inability of your body to properly convert the food that you eat into energy to fuel your cells. People with the MD Factor have difficulty regulating their blood sugar, which is often due to insulin resistance or even diabetes. In both instances, their bodies are unable to pull glucose into the cells, which means that excess levels of

glucose build up in the blood. With nowhere else to go, the body turns this extra energy into fat and stores it for later.

This infographic outlines the symptoms and causes of insulin resistance, or metabolism dysfunction.

Surprisingly, you don't have to be overweight for your cells to be insulin-resistant. Even if your weight is perfectly normal, you can still suffer from its effects. Metabolism dysfunction doesn't develop overnight and could be caused by one or more triggers including: aging and menopause, genetics, belly/visceral fat, medications, and nutritional deficiencies. We'll cover all these in subsequent posts. But for now, we'll cover the two reasons you have no control over -- genetic predisposition and aging.

DNA has a big impact on your weight (The MD Factor Diet, 2015). When I was in medical school I read an article that made a lasting impression. It said that if both parents were obese, the child had an 80 percent likelihood of becoming obese. This struck me not only because it's a staggering statistic, but because my family has always suffered with our weight, I have to be very mindful of my own diet and exercise because I'm genetically predisposed to gain and retain weight.

You may have been born with cells that don't respond well to insulin. If your family has a history of diabetes (particularly from your parents) you're at high risk of developing a dysfunctional metabolism. Your genes also determine how your body stores fat (e.g., if you're apple-shaped, you'll carry fat in your abdominal area and be at risk of having two contributing factors genetics and belly fat to your Insulin Resistance).

Just like we can't control the genes we were born with, we all grow older. As this occurs, our hormones gradually decline. Declining hormone levels affect muscle mass causing it to be lost first while your body holds onto its fat stores. As you age, you need to be more mindful of what you eat and your physical lifestyle. After all, few of us can eat the same at 50 as we did at 30.

There are several examples of correlation of aging and weight. Pre-menopausal women typically gain 10-15 pounds (though I've had patients with up to 30-pound weight gain) around menopause (Women's Health Research Program, Department of Epidemiology and Preventive Medicine, Monash University, Melbourne, Australia). It's not just hormones like testosterone and estrogen that shift to affect your weight. The body's ability to use insulin does gradually decline, though it can be slowed by diet and regular physical activity. Type 2 diabetes has been shown to get more prevalent as you age, according to the Centers for Disease Control. Currently, half of all Americans aged 65 years and older have prediabetes. Without lifestyle changes to improve their health and manage Insulin Resistance, up to 30 percent of people with prediabetes will develop Type 2 diabetes within five years.

In order to avoid weight gain, diabetes, and other medical problems (like heart disease) as you age, you need to eat and exercise to minimize the effects of insulin resistance.

Do you have a dysfunctional metabolism?

My patients feel a lot better about their weight struggles once they realize that they're overweight not because they ate too much or are lazy. Body weight and weight regulation are highly complex and influenced by many different genes. You may have been born with factors out of your control, but you can put that control back in your capable hands.

Take this free quiz to see if you have sensitivities to insulin, and get an action plan featuring what steps you can take to start correcting your metabolism dysfunction:

Insulin resistance is caused by changes in how your body is able to use the nutrients in your food. It's very common, but not often recognized by those who have it or their physicians.

If you've tried to lose weight and haven't made any real progress, one thing is certain: Your metabolism has changed. Your old metabolism has been replaced by one that likes storing fat.

Healthy lifestyle and diet is important and can help regulate insulin levels. Exercise can also help the body regulate blood glucose and keep excess weight off.

You may have been born with genetic predisposition to gain and retain weight, but by making a few lifestyle changes, you can reverse the impact of the MD factor. By adjusting your diet and lifestyle, you can eat better, sleep better, have more energy, be sharper and more focused and lower your risk for heart disease, some cancers, stroke and dementia.

5 WAYS TO PREVENT INSULIN RESISTANCE AND DIABETES

Insulin resistance has become one of the most widespread health problems in America. High-stress lifestyles, consuming too much fast food or chemical laden, high-carb processed foods, and lack of exercise has created an epidemic of insulin resistance and Type 2 Diabetes. But you don't have to be one of those statistics.

Adopting these five simple lifestyle and diet changes corrects the problems that cause insulin resistance. If you are already insulin resistant, these five changes can prevent your condition from deteriorating into Type 2 Diabetes. And if you have already been diagnosed as a diabetic, it's still not too late to control blood sugar levels and improve your health with these vital five steps. Though each person is different, it is even possible for some people to reverse diabetes and restore normal pancreatic functions using these five steps.

1: Exercise!

30 minutes of brisk walking or similar exercise, 3-5 times a week, can prevent you developing insulin resistance or diabetes. If you're already insulin resistant or diabetic, exercise will help improve insulin sensitivity and lower blood sugar levels.

2. Avoid processed foods.

Packaged and processed foods contain two things that can lead to insulin resistance and eventually diabetes: high-fructose corn syrup and trans fats.

High fructose corn syrup is a chemically altered sugar that your body cannot use, but your pancreas still detects it as the presence of sugar and attempts to process it by releasing insulin. Consuming too much of it contributes to weight gain, hypertension (high blood pressure) and Type 2 Diabetes. This insidious stuff is in absolutely everything even foods that you wouldn't suspect of containing sugar, such as crackers, salad dressings even tomato sauce! Non-diet soft drinks and virtually all commercially packaged juices contain high levels of fructose corn syrup.

Trans fats are notorious for causing inflammation in the arteries and other problems. They also seem to contribute to the onset of diabetes, though how is not entirely understood. You'll find trans fat in most packaged cake and frosting mixes, many cookies and other baked products, non-dairy coffee creamers, and margarines. Virtually all "stick" type margarines contain trans fat check the label, and you'll see. Your body cannot metabolize these chemically altered fats, which simply build up in your tissues, damaging cells and contributing to life-threatening arterial blockage.

3. Eat more whole grains, fresh fruits and veggies

Along with contributing important nutrients and

aiding digestion, these foods can help to stabilize blood sugar and insulin levels by slowing down your digestive process. Unlike "simple" carbohydrates like white bread, potatoes and pasta which quickly break down into sugar, causing your blood sugar levels to soar and insulin levels to spike these more complex foods digest more slowly, causing sugar to be released more gradually into your blood, avoiding the destructive "sugar spikes" that come from eating starchy foods.

4. Add the "right" fats to your diet

Not all fats are "bad". In fact, fat is an essential nutrient which your body needs. The key is making sure the fat you add to your diet is the right kind of fat. Unlike synthetic or chemically altered "trans fats" or "hydrogenated fats", your body can digest "natural" fats, such as mono and poly-unsaturated vegetable oils. Fats and oils high in "essential fatty acids" (EFAs), such as those found in salmon, tuna and avocados help reduce "bad" cholesterol levels and raise "good" cholesterol levels. Flax seed oil is another beneficial source of fat, as are those found in nuts. In addition to fats, nuts and flax seed add other valuable nutrients to your dietary mix.

5. Add important nutrients to your diet

It's difficult for us to get sufficient nutrients from food alone because processing strips food of nutrients, and because today's mass-production farming methods result in soil that is "depleted" of important minerals and vitamins. A good multi-vitamin/mineral supplement can help to solve this problem. But if you are insulin resistant or diabetic, you should be sure that your supplement contains certain trace elements and vitamins that have been shown to help control blood sugar and lower insulin levels. These include:

Chromium - in the form of chromium picolinate, it helps control blood sugar and insulin levels

Magnesium - this is the nutrient that most often seems to be lacking in both Type 1 and Type 2 diabetics, so evidence is strong that a lack of this trace mineral in your diet can be a determining factor in whether or not you develop diabetes, regardless of family history, lack of exercise, etc.

Manganese - its role in preventing diabetes and insulin resistance is stll being researched, but lower than normal levels of manganese are another thing most diabetics seem to have in common, so it would stand to reason that getting adequate levels in a daily supplement might help to prevent the onset of diabetes.

Vanadium - aids in the metabolism of sugar and increases the insulin sensitivity of cells

B Vitamins - Stress can deplete your body of all-important B-viatmins and cause blood sugar levels to rise.

B3 (Niacin) - is valuable for circulatory health, and also key to metabolizing carbs, fat and protein.

B6 - this powerful antioxidant helps protect you from the destructive effects of diabetes like nerve and heart damage.

B12 - vital to the proper functioning of nerve cells, B12 is another good anti-stress nutrient, and may actually help prevent the nerve damage associated with diabetes

INSULIN RESISTANCE DIET SHOPPING LIST

Since I started on this lifestyle in progress, my shopping needs have changed. I remember pushing a shopping trolley at the green grocer's and noticing the colour of the contents. It was mostly green.

My pantry has previously been cleared of unsuitable items and now holds mostly condiments such as sauces and spices. My fridge is full of fresh vegetables and herbs. My freezer holds meat, fish, chicken and seafood at times.

To make it easier to shop every week, I have compiled this Insulin Resistance Diet Shopping List divided into Supermarket, Green Grocer, Deli Items, Protein and Miscellaneous. I hope you will find it useful.

Supermarket Shopping List

- ✓ Canola vegetable oil
- ✓ Capers
- ✓ Coconut milk, low fat
- ✓ Dijon mustard
- ✓ Dried Herbs and Spices: chilli powder, chilli flakes, dried oregano, turmeric, cayenne pepper, cumin powder, smoked paprika, bouquet garni, nutmeg, black peppercorns, sea salt, bay leaves, cinnamon, ground coriander seed, black peppercorns
- ✓ Eggs

- ✓ Fish sauce, nam pla
- ✓ Frozen berries
- ✓ Green tea
- ✓ Miso soup
- ✓ Olive oil
- ✓ Oyster sauce
- ✓ Passata
- ✓ Red Thai curry paste
- ✓ Red wine vinegar
- ✓ Sesame oil
- ✓ Soy sauce
- ✓ Stock: vegetable, chicken, beef, fish (low salt)
- ✓ Supermarket
- ✓ Tabasco sauce
- ✓ Tahini
- ✓ Thai curry paste – green and red
- ✓ Tinned tomatoes – make sure they have no added sugar
- ✓ Tinned tuna
- ✓ Tomato juice – no added sugar variety
- ✓ Tomato paste – check for the lowest carb/sugar content
- ✓ Vegemite
- ✓ Wasabi
- ✓ Worcestershire sauce

Green Grocer Shopping List

- ✓ Baby Spinach
- ✓ Berries (strawberries, blueberries, raspberries)
- ✓ Boy choy

- ✓ Broccoli
- ✓ Carrots
- ✓ Cauliflower
- ✓ Celery
- ✓ Chilli peppers
- ✓ Choy sum
- ✓ Cucumber
- ✓ Eggplant
- ✓ Fennel
- ✓ Garlic
- ✓ Ginger
- ✓ Green beans
- ✓ Herbs: parsley, coriander, chives, thyme, basil, dill, rosemary
- ✓ Lemon
- ✓ Lime
- ✓ Mixed lettuce leaves
- ✓ Mushrooms
- ✓ Natural almonds
- ✓ Onion
- ✓ Red/green peppers (capsicum)
- ✓ Savoy Cabbage
- ✓ Shallots
- ✓ Snow peas
- ✓ Spanish onion
- ✓ Tomatoes
- ✓ Zucchini
- ✓ Protein Shopping List
- ✓ Beef – lean mince, lean steak
- ✓ Chicken – organic or free range whole chicken or chicken breasts

- ✓ Pink fish – salmon, ocean trout, smoked salmon, hot-smoked salmon, tuna
- ✓ Seafood – green prawns, oysters, crab claws, mussels, squid
- ✓ White fish – ling, snapper, barramundi, cod
- ✓ Delicatessen Shopping List
- ✓ Basturma – air dried beef
- ✓ Cheese – aged cheddar, Parmesan, goats cheese, bocconcini, blue cheese
- ✓ Ham – off the bone or gypsy ham
- ✓ Olives – black or green
- ✓ Miscellaneous Items
- ✓ Coffee beans
- ✓ Sourdough bread

THE BEST SUPPLEMENTS FOR INSULIN RESISTANCE

The hormone insulin stimulates body tissues to absorb blood sugar, and then burn it for fuel or store it for later use. Insulin resistance is a condition in which the body gradually loses its ability to use insulin effectively. To compensate, excess amounts of insulin are produced and released into the bloodstream. Insulin resistance is the primary metabolic abnormality that leads to pre-diabetes and type 2 diabetes (T2DM). Certain nutritional supplements such as chromium, alpha-lipoic acid, omega-3 fatty acids, zinc and magnesium might help reduce insulin resistance, leading to more efficient use of insulin.

Different pills and capsules in glass jar on white background.

Volume 30%

- ✓ 00:15
- ✓ 00:10
- ✓ 00:38

Chromium

Chromium is a trace mineral the body requires to process fats and carbohydrates. It works through complex mechanisms to boost the effectiveness of insulin in body tissue. A March 2014 "Journal of

Clinical Pharmacy and Therapeutics" review article pooled results from 22 studies to determine the effects of chromium supplementation on blood sugar and fat levels in people with diabetes. People taking a daily chromium picolinate supplement had lower fasting blood sugar levels, compared to those not taking chromium. Among people with poor blood sugar control, daily supplementation with at least 200 micrograms of chromium was also found to lower A1C, a measure of blood sugar over three months. This effect was seen in people taking chromium picolinate or brewer's yeast, but not in those taking chromium yeast or chromium dinicocysteinate.

In examining the effects of chromium supplementation on blood fat levels, the researchers found no reduction in total cholesterol or LDL, the "bad"

form of cholesterol. However, people taking chromium picolinate experienced a significant decrease in triglycerides and increased HDL, the "good" form of cholesterol.

Alpha-Lipoic Acid

Alpha-lipoic acid (ALA) is an antioxidant naturally produced by the body. Like other antioxidants, ALA neutralizes potentially harmful substances called free radicals. An overabundance of free radicals, known as oxidative stress, is thought to be a factor in the development and progression of diabetes and its associated complications. Some research suggests that oxidative stress may also contribute to insulin resistance. This has led to interest in using supplemental ALA as a possible way to counteract insulin resistance.

Although the effectiveness of oral ALA remains to be conclusively proven, a small eight-week study reported in the June 2011 issue of "Saudi Medical Journal" found that 300 mg of ALA daily significantly lowered insulin resistance and fasting blood sugar. The authors noted their findings were consistent with animal and laboratory experiments, and at least two other small studies on humans. While these results are promising, additional research is needed to confirm whether oral ALA is beneficial for people with diabetes.

Omega-3 Fatty Acids

Omega-3 fatty acids abundant in fish oil, some vegetable oils and nuts are best known for their role in heart disease prevention. This is important because diabetes increases heart disease risk. In addition, a December 2011 "Clinical Nutrition" article that reviewed the research on omega-3 fatty acids said they may help reduce insulin resistance, although some studies have found no effect. For example, a July 2008 "Diabetologia" article found that fish oil supplementation during a two-month weight-loss program among overweight adults led to greater improvements in insulin sensitivity, compared to those not taking the supplement. However, a December 2007 "American Journal of Clinical Nutrition" article found two

months of daily fish oil supplementation did not improve insulin sensitivity among women with T2DM.

Omega-3 fatty acids have many effects in the body, but how they might affect insulin resistance isn't entirely understood. Omega-3s reduce triglycerides, suppress fat production in the liver, and help liver and muscle tissue burn fat. It is believed that these effects and others can potentially improve insulin sensitivity. People who take blood thinners should consult with their healthcare provider before taking omega-3 fatty acid supplements, because these can prolong bleeding time.

Magnesium

Magnesium is an essential nutrient that has crucial roles in insulin secretion and metabolism of blood glucose. Low magnesium levels are common in people with T2DM, because of decreased intake and increased loss through the urine. Magnesium plays a complex role in enabling insulin usage, and insufficient magnesium may be a contributing factor to insulin resistance.

The relationship of magnesium to insulin resistance was examined in a study published in the October 2013 issue of the journal "Nutrients." The study included 234 adults with metabolic syndrome, a condition associated with increased risk for T2DM and heart disease. The researchers found that those who had the largest dietary intake of magnesium were 71 percent less likely to experience insulin resistance, compared to those with the lowest intake of magnesium. Another study published in April 2003 in "Diabetes Care" found that 16 weeks of oral magnesium supplementation improved insulin sensitivity among people with T2DM who were magnesium-deficient.

Zinc

Zinc is another essential nutrient that influences critical functions involving insulin production and release, and its effects on body tissue. Zinc deficiency is associated with insulin resistance and increased blood sugar. Zinc works both independently and in combination with insulin to enhance

glucose absorption from the bloodstream into the cells of the body. Zinc is also necessary for effective insulin release from the pancreas, and helps protect insulin-producing cells from damage caused by oxidative stress.

In a small study among obese women without diabetes, supplementation with 30 mg of zinc daily decreased insulin resistance, as reported in the June 2012 issue of "Nutrition Research and Practice." Another study reported in December 2010 in "Metabolic Syndrome and Related Disorders" also found improved insulin sensitivity among obese children after eight weeks of zinc supplementation. An April 2012 "Diabetology and Metabolic Syndrome" article that reported on the effects of zinc supplementation for diabetes evaluated pooled results from 25 studies, including 22 among people with T2DM. The researchers reported that zinc supplementation was found to lower blood sugar levels, although insulin resistance was not directly measured.

A healthy eating plan, exercise and losing excess weight are the cornerstones of treatment for insulin resistance that has not yet progressed to T2DM. Medication called metformin (Glucophage, Fortamet, Glumetza) is also sometimes prescribed. Other medications are often used for people with T2DM.

The potential role of nutritional supplements for insulin resistance treatment is still being investigated. As of 2016, the American Diabetes Association does not recommend nutritional supplements for treatment of pre-diabetes or T2DM. Many people, however, opt to use supplements as part of their treatment plan. If you're interested in adding supplements to your regimen, talk with your healthcare provider. This is important because supplements can interact with medications, including diabetes medications. Some nutritional supplements might also cause potentially dangerous side effects. Regular blood sugar monitoring is essential if you're taking supplements along with diabetes medications. Adjustments in diabetes medication dosages might be necessary, but you should never stop taking your medicines or change the dosages unless your doctor instructs you to do so.

5 WAYS TO DECREASE INSULIN RESISTANCE

Insulin resistance disrupts our ability to effectively regulate our sugar intake. This can lead to health problems such as obesity, metabolic syndrome, and diabetes. Read on to discover 5 ways you can decrease insulin resistance.

Insulin Resistance And Poor Health

The problem isn't insulin, but rather insulin resistance. If you are insulin resistant your brain will not get the message that insulin is trying hard to convey (that you have high levels of sugar in your bloodstream).

In this way, insulin resistance promotes hunger. You eat and insulin is released, but your body tells you to eat some more despite the ability of insulin to act as a satiety hormone. Hence why obesity is linked to brain insulin resistance.

When rats had their brain insulin receptors removed, they ate more, developed insulin resistance, and became obese. There is a correlation between insulin resistance and fat accumulation in the liver.

Insulin resistance was shown to be directly correlated to non-alcoholic fatty liver disease in a literature review.

Elevated blood free fatty acids (FFA) were shown to cause insulin resistance.

In diabetics, insulin resistance was shown to severely inhibit a marker for muscular performance (glycogen synthesis and uptake). Also, waist and thigh circumference (predictors of insulin resistance) were negatively correlated with the percentage of type 1 muscle fibers.

When rats were fed a high-fat diet insulin resistance occurred first in fat and liver tissue than in muscle tissue.

In prediabetic subjects, insulin resistance was linked to atherogenic changes TNF-a levels were linked to the development of insulin resistance in obese patients. TNF-a was shown to inhibit the ability of insulin to exert its effects on the insulin receptor .

IKKB (a mediator of inflammatory cytokine Nf-kb production) has been linked to the development of insulin resistance.

Anti-inflammatory cytokine (IL-10) is able to counter the insulin resistance caused by inflammatory cytokine.

Insulin is able to induce the secretion of an inflammatory marker (MCP-1), which may contribute to many diseases associated with hyperinsulinemia.

Leptin was shown in rats to increase insulin sensitivity. Leptin inhibits the ability of insulin to cause glucose uptake and fat synthesis in fatty tissue.

In individuals with low levels of HGH (human growth hormone) supplementation of rHGH was able to lower insulin sensitivity.

There is a direct correlation between insulin resistance and chronic kidney disease patholog.

Methods for Decreasing Insulin Resistance

Weight Loss

Weight loss has been shown to improve insulin sensitivity.

If you are overweight, the single most important thing you can do is lose weight.

Exercise

In a literature review, high-intensity interval exercise (like sprints) was correlated with greater insulin sensitivity.

Exercise without weight loss showed improvements in insulin resistance in sedentary adults.

Moderate Alcohol Consumption

In postmenopausal women, moderate consumption of alcohol (30g per day) was associated with greater insulin sensitivity.

Resistant Starch

In ten healthy subjects supplementation of resistant starch was able to increase insulin sensitivity,

- ✓ Vitamins and Minerals
- ✓ Vitamin D3,
- ✓ K2,
- ✓ Zinc,
- ✓ Magnesium,
- ✓ GTF Chromium,
- ✓ Calcium Citrate.
- ✓ Other Supplements
- ✓ Hi-maize resistant starch
- ✓ Kombucha tea, Bragg Apple Cider Vinegar or Apple Cider Vinegar
- ✓ Grape Seed Extract
- ✓ Ceylon Cinnamon

Berberine – These supplements are good for overweight and thin people

Inositol

5 WAYS TO PREVENT INSULIN RESISTANCE AND DIABETES

Insulin resistance has become one of the most widespread health problems in America. High-stress lifestyles, consuming too much fast food or chemical laden, high-carb processed foods, and lack of exercise has created an epidemic of insulin resistance and Type 2 Diabetes. But you don't have to be one of those statistics.

Adopting these five simple lifestyle and diet changes corrects the problems that cause insulin resistance. If you are already insulin resistant, these five changes can prevent your condition from deteriorating into Type 2 Diabetes. And if you have already been diagnosed as a diabetic, it's still not too late to control blood sugar levels and improve your health with these vital five steps. Though each person is different, it is even possible for some people to reverse diabetes and restore normal pancreatic functions using these five steps.

1: Exercise!

30 minutes of brisk walking or similar exercise, 3-5 times a week, can prevent you developing insulin resistance or diabetes. If you're already insulin resistant or diabetic, exercise will help improve insulin sensitivity and lower blood sugar levels.

2. Avoid processed foods.

Packaged and processed foods contain two things that can lead to insulin resistance and eventually diabetes: high-fructose corn syrup and trans fats.

High fructose corn syrup is a chemically altered sugar that your body cannot use, but your pancreas still detects it as the presence of sugar and attempts to process it by releasing insulin. Consuming too much of it contributes to weight gain, hypertension (high blood pressure) and Type 2 Diabetes. This insidious stuff is in absolutely everything even foods that you wouldn't suspect of containing sugar, such as crackers, salad dressings even tomato sauce! Non-diet soft drinks and virtually all commercially packaged juices contain high levels of fructose corn syrup.

Trans fats are notorious for causing inflammation in the arteries and other problems. They also seem to contribute to the onset of diabetes, though how is not entirely understood. You'll find trans fat in most packaged cake and frosting mixes, many cookies and other baked products, non-dairy coffee creamers, and margarines. Virtually all "stick" type margarines contain trans fat check the label, and you'll see. Your body cannot metabolize these chemically altered fats, which simply build up in your tissues, damaging cells and contributing to life-threatening arterial blockage.

3. Eat more whole grains, fresh fruits and veggies

Along with contributing important nutrients and aiding digestion, these foods can help to stabilize blood sugar and insulin levels by slowing down your digestive process. Unlike "simple" carbohydrates like white bread, potatoes and pasta which quickly break down into sugar, causing your blood sugar levels to soar and insulin levels to spike these more complex foods digest more slowly, causing sugar to be released more gradually into your blood, avoiding the destructive "sugar spikes" that come from eating starchy foods.

4. Add the "right" fats to your diet

Not all fats are "bad". In fact, fat is an essential nutrient which your body needs. The key is making sure the fat you add to your diet is the right kind of fat. Unlike synthetic or chemically altered "trans fats" or "hydrogenated fats", your body can digest "natural" fats, such as mono and poly-unsaturated vegetable oils. Fats and oils high in "essential fatty acids" (EFAs), such as those found in salmon, tuna and avocados help reduce "bad" cholesterol levels and raise "good" cholesterol levels. Flax seed oil is another beneficial source of fat, as are those found in nuts. In addition to fats, nuts and flax seed add other valuable nutrients to your dietary mix.

5. Add important nutrients to your diet

It's difficult for us to get sufficient nutrients from food alone because processing strips food of nutrients, and because today's mass-production farming methods result in soil that is "depleted" of important minerals and vitamins. A good multi-vitamin/mineral supplement can help to solve this problem. But if you are insulin resistant or diabetic, you should be sure that your supplement contains certain trace elements and vitamins that have been shown to help control blood sugar and lower insulin levels. These include:

Chromium - in the form of chromium picolinate, it helps control blood sugar and insulin levels

Magnesium - this is the nutrient that most often seems to be lacking in both Type 1 and Type 2 diabetics, so evidence is strong that a lack of this trace mineral in your diet can be a determining factor in whether or not you develop diabetes, regardless of family history, lack of exercise, etc.

Manganese - its role in preventing diabetes and insulin resistance is stll being researched, but lower than normal levels of manganese are another thing most diabetics seem to have in common, so it would stand to reason that getting adequate levels in a daily supplement might help to prevent the onset of diabetes.

Vanadium - aids in the metabolism of sugar and increases the insulin sensitivity of cells

B Vitamins - Stress can deplete your body of all-important B-viatmins and cause blood sugar levels to rise.

B3 (Niacin) - is valuable for circulatory health, and also key to metabolizing carbs, fat and protein.

B6 - this powerful antioxidant helps protect you from the destructive effects of diabetes like nerve and heart damage.

B12 - vital to the proper functioning of nerve cells, B12 is another good anti-stress nutrient, and may actually help prevent the nerve damage associated with diabetes

INSULIN RESISTANCE DIET SHOPPING LIST

Since I started on this lifestyle in progress, my shopping needs have changed. I remember pushing a shopping trolley at the green grocer's and noticing the colour of the contents. It was mostly green.

My pantry has previously been cleared of unsuitable items and now holds mostly condiments such as sauces and spices. My fridge is full of fresh vegetables and herbs. My freezer holds meat, fish, chicken and seafood at times.

To make it easier to shop every week, I have compiled this Insulin Resistance Diet Shopping List divided into Supermarket, Green Grocer, Deli Items, Protein and Miscellaneous. I hope you will find it useful.

Supermarket Shopping List

- ✓ Canola vegetable oil
- ✓ Capers
- ✓ Coconut milk, low fat
- ✓ Dijon mustard
- ✓ Dried Herbs and Spices: chilli powder, chilli flakes, dried oregano, turmeric, cayenne pepper, cumin powder, smoked paprika, bouquet garni, nutmeg, black peppercorns, sea salt, bay leaves, cinnamon, ground coriander seed, black peppercorns

- ✓ Eggs
- ✓ Fish sauce, nam pla
- ✓ Frozen berries
- ✓ Green tea
- ✓ Miso soup
- ✓ Olive oil
- ✓ Oyster sauce
- ✓ Passata
- ✓ Red Thai curry paste
- ✓ Red wine vinegar
- ✓ Sesame oil
- ✓ Soy sauce
- ✓ Stock: vegetable, chicken, beef, fish (low salt)
- ✓ Supermarket
- ✓ Tabasco sauce
- ✓ Tahini
- ✓ Thai curry paste – green and red
- ✓ Tinned tomatoes – make sure they have no added sugar
- ✓ Tinned tuna
- ✓ Tomato juice – no added sugar variety
- ✓ Tomato paste – check for the lowest carb/sugar content
- ✓ Vegemite
- ✓ Wasabi
- ✓ Worcestershire sauce

Green Grocer Shopping List

- ✓ Baby Spinach
- ✓ Berries (strawberries, blueberries, raspberries)

- ✓ Boy choy
- ✓ Broccoli
- ✓ Carrots
- ✓ Cauliflower
- ✓ Celery
- ✓ Chilli peppers
- ✓ Choy sum
- ✓ Cucumber
- ✓ Eggplant
- ✓ Fennel
- ✓ Garlic
- ✓ Ginger
- ✓ Green beans
- ✓ Herbs: parsley, coriander, chives, thyme, basil, dill, rosemary
- ✓ Lemon
- ✓ Lime
- ✓ Mixed lettuce leaves
- ✓ Mushrooms
- ✓ Natural almonds
- ✓ Onion
- ✓ Red/green peppers (capsicum)
- ✓ Savoy Cabbage
- ✓ Shallots
- ✓ Snow peas
- ✓ Spanish onion
- ✓ Tomatoes
- ✓ Zucchini
- ✓ Protein Shopping List
- ✓ Beef – lean mince, lean steak

- ✓ Chicken – organic or free range whole chicken or chicken breasts
- ✓ Pink fish – salmon, ocean trout, smoked salmon, hot-smoked salmon, tuna
- ✓ Seafood – green prawns, oysters, crab claws, mussels, squid
- ✓ White fish – ling, snapper, barramundi, cod
- ✓ Delicatessen Shopping List
- ✓ Basturma – air dried beef
- ✓ Cheese – aged cheddar, Parmesan, goats cheese, bocconcini, blue cheese
- ✓ Ham – off the bone or gypsy ham
- ✓ Olives – black or green
- ✓ Miscellaneous Items
- ✓ Coffee beans
- ✓ Sourdough bread

THE BEST SUPPLEMENTS FOR INSULIN RESISTANCE

The hormone insulin stimulates body tissues to absorb blood sugar, and then burn it for fuel or store it for later use. Insulin resistance is a condition in which the body gradually loses its ability to use insulin effectively. To compensate, excess amounts of insulin are produced and released into the bloodstream. Insulin resistance is the primary metabolic abnormality that leads to pre-diabetes and type 2 diabetes (T2DM). Certain nutritional supplements such as chromium, alpha-lipoic acid, omega-3 fatty acids, zinc and magnesium might help reduce insulin resistance, leading to more efficient use of insulin.

Different pills and capsules in glass jar on white background.

Volume 30%

- ✓ 00:15
- ✓ 00:10
- ✓ 00:38

Chromium

Chromium is a trace mineral the body requires to process fats and carbohydrates. It works through complex mechanisms to boost the effectiveness of insulin in body tissue. A March 2014 "Journal of

Clinical Pharmacy and Therapeutics" review article pooled results from 22 studies to determine the effects of chromium supplementation on blood sugar and fat levels in people with diabetes. People taking a daily chromium picolinate supplement had lower fasting blood sugar levels, compared to those not taking chromium. Among people with poor blood sugar control, daily supplementation with at least 200 micrograms of chromium was also found to lower A1C, a measure of blood sugar over three months. This effect was seen in people taking chromium picolinate or brewer's yeast, but not in those taking chromium yeast or chromium dinicocysteinate.

In examining the effects of chromium supplementation on blood fat levels, the researchers found no reduction in total cholesterol or LDL, the "bad"

form of cholesterol. However, people taking chromium picolinate experienced a significant decrease in triglycerides and increased HDL, the "good" form of cholesterol.

Alpha-Lipoic Acid

Alpha-lipoic acid (ALA) is an antioxidant naturally produced by the body. Like other antioxidants, ALA neutralizes potentially harmful substances called free radicals. An overabundance of free radicals, known as oxidative stress, is thought to be a factor in the development and progression of diabetes and its associated complications. Some research suggests that oxidative stress may also contribute to insulin resistance. This has led to interest in using supplemental ALA as a possible way to counteract insulin resistance.

Although the effectiveness of oral ALA remains to be conclusively proven, a small eight-week study reported in the June 2011 issue of "Saudi Medical Journal" found that 300 mg of ALA daily significantly lowered insulin resistance and fasting blood sugar. The authors noted their findings were consistent with animal and laboratory experiments, and at least two other small studies on humans. While these results are promising, additional research is needed to confirm whether oral ALA is beneficial for people with diabetes.

Omega-3 Fatty Acids

Omega-3 fatty acids abundant in fish oil, some vegetable oils and nuts are best known for their role in heart disease prevention. This is important because diabetes increases heart disease risk. In addition, a December 2011 "Clinical Nutrition" article that reviewed the research on omega-3 fatty acids said they may help reduce insulin resistance, although some studies have found no effect. For example, a July 2008 "Diabetologia" article found that fish oil supplementation during a two-month weight-loss program among overweight adults led to greater improvements in insulin sensitivity, compared to those not taking the supplement. However, a December 2007 "American Journal of Clinical Nutrition" article found two

months of daily fish oil supplementation did not improve insulin sensitivity among women with T2DM.

Omega-3 fatty acids have many effects in the body, but how they might affect insulin resistance isn't entirely understood. Omega-3s reduce triglycerides, suppress fat production in the liver, and help liver and muscle tissue burn fat. It is believed that these effects and others can potentially improve insulin sensitivity. People who take blood thinners should consult with their healthcare provider before taking omega-3 fatty acid supplements, because these can prolong bleeding time.

Magnesium

Magnesium is an essential nutrient that has crucial roles in insulin secretion and metabolism of blood glucose. Low magnesium levels are common in people with T2DM, because of decreased intake and increased loss through the urine. Magnesium plays a complex role in enabling insulin usage, and insufficient magnesium may be a contributing factor to insulin resistance.

The relationship of magnesium to insulin resistance was examined in a study published in the October 2013 issue of the journal "Nutrients." The study included 234 adults with metabolic syndrome, a condition associated with increased risk for T2DM and heart disease. The researchers found that those who had the largest dietary intake of magnesium were 71 percent less likely to experience insulin resistance, compared to those with the lowest intake of magnesium. Another study published in April 2003 in "Diabetes Care" found that 16 weeks of oral magnesium supplementation improved insulin sensitivity among people with T2DM who were magnesium-deficient.

Zinc

Zinc is another essential nutrient that influences critical functions involving insulin production and release, and its effects on body tissue. Zinc deficiency is associated with insulin resistance and increased blood sugar. Zinc works both independently and in combination with insulin to enhance

glucose absorption from the bloodstream into the cells of the body. Zinc is also necessary for effective insulin release from the pancreas, and helps protect insulin-producing cells from damage caused by oxidative stress.

In a small study among obese women without diabetes, supplementation with 30 mg of zinc daily decreased insulin resistance, as reported in the June 2012 issue of "Nutrition Research and Practice." Another study reported in December 2010 in "Metabolic Syndrome and Related Disorders" also found improved insulin sensitivity among obese children after eight weeks of zinc supplementation. An April 2012 "Diabetology and Metabolic Syndrome" article that reported on the effects of zinc supplementation for diabetes evaluated pooled results from 25 studies, including 22 among people with T2DM. The researchers reported that zinc supplementation was found to lower blood sugar levels, although insulin resistance was not directly measured.

A healthy eating plan, exercise and losing excess weight are the cornerstones of treatment for insulin resistance that has not yet progressed to T2DM. Medication called metformin (Glucophage, Fortamet, Glumetza) is also sometimes prescribed. Other medications are often used for people with T2DM.

The potential role of nutritional supplements for insulin resistance treatment is still being investigated. As of 2016, the American Diabetes Association does not recommend nutritional supplements for treatment of pre-diabetes or T2DM. Many people, however, opt to use supplements as part of their treatment plan. If you're interested in adding supplements to your regimen, talk with your healthcare provider. This is important because supplements can interact with medications, including diabetes medications. Some nutritional supplements might also cause potentially dangerous side effects. Regular blood sugar monitoring is essential if you're taking supplements along with diabetes medications. Adjustments in diabetes medication dosages might be necessary, but you should never stop taking your medicines or change the dosages unless your doctor instructs you to do so.

5 WAYS TO DECREASE INSULIN RESISTANCE

Insulin resistance disrupts our ability to effectively regulate our sugar intake. This can lead to health problems such as obesity, metabolic syndrome, and diabetes. Read on to discover 5 ways you can decrease insulin resistance.

Insulin Resistance And Poor Health

The problem isn't insulin, but rather insulin resistance. If you are insulin resistant your brain will not get the message that insulin is trying hard to convey (that you have high levels of sugar in your bloodstream).

In this way, insulin resistance promotes hunger. You eat and insulin is released, but your body tells you to eat some more despite the ability of insulin to act as a satiety hormone. Hence why obesity is linked to brain insulin resistance.

When rats had their brain insulin receptors removed, they ate more, developed insulin resistance, and became obese. There is a correlation between insulin resistance and fat accumulation in the liver.

Insulin resistance was shown to be directly correlated to non-alcoholic fatty liver disease in a literature review.

Elevated blood free fatty acids (FFA) were shown to cause insulin resistance.

In diabetics, insulin resistance was shown to severely inhibit a marker for muscular performance (glycogen synthesis and uptake). Also, waist and thigh circumference (predictors of insulin resistance) were negatively correlated with the percentage of type 1 muscle fibers.

When rats were fed a high-fat diet insulin resistance occurred first in fat and liver tissue than in muscle tissue.

In prediabetic subjects, insulin resistance was linked to atherogenic changes TNF-a levels were linked to the development of insulin resistance in obese patients. TNF-a was shown to inhibit the ability of insulin to exert its effects on the insulin receptor .

IKKB (a mediator of inflammatory cytokine Nf-kb production) has been linked to the development of insulin resistance.

Anti-inflammatory cytokine (IL-10) is able to counter the insulin resistance caused by inflammatory cytokine.

Insulin is able to induce the secretion of an inflammatory marker (MCP-1), which may contribute to many diseases associated with hyperinsulinemia.

Leptin was shown in rats to increase insulin sensitivity.

Leptin inhibits the ability of insulin to cause glucose uptake and fat synthesis in fatty tissue.

In individuals with low levels of HGH (human growth hormone) supplementation of rHGH was able to lower insulin sensitivity.

There is a direct correlation between insulin resistance and chronic kidney disease patholog.

Methods for Decreasing Insulin Resistance

Weight Loss

Weight loss has been shown to improve insulin sensitivity.

If you are overweight, the single most important thing you can do is lose weight.

Exercise

In a literature review, high-intensity interval exercise (like sprints) was correlated with greater insulin sensitivity.

Exercise without weight loss showed improvements in insulin resistance in sedentary adults.

Moderate Alcohol Consumption

In postmenopausal women, moderate consumption of alcohol (30g per day) was associated with greater insulin sensitivity.

Resistant Starch

In ten healthy subjects supplementation of resistant starch was able to increase insulin sensitivity,

- ✓ Vitamins and Minerals
- ✓ Vitamin D3,
- ✓ K2,
- ✓ Zinc,
- ✓ Magnesium,
- ✓ GTF Chromium,
- ✓ Calcium Citrate.
- ✓ Other Supplements
- ✓ Hi-maize resistant starch
- ✓ Kombucha tea, Bragg Apple Cider Vinegar or Apple Cider Vinegar
- ✓ Grape Seed Extract
- ✓ Ceylon Cinnamon

Berberine – These supplements are good for overweight and thin people

Inositol

CONCLUSION

Insulin resistance and the diseases associated with it represent major public health challenges in the United States and around the world. Although it would be attractive to find an ideal diet for the prevention and treatment of insulin resistance states, this is probably an unrealistic expectation. Knowledge gained from both animal and human studies about the effect of simple and complex carbohydrates on insulin action is increasing. However, any change in the carbohydrate composition of the diet may produce reciprocal changes in other parts of the diet.

It is important to remember that on balance, increased energy intake and positive energy balance may be the nutritional factors that are most to blame for insulin resistance through the production of obesity. In addition, energy restriction, independent of the composition of the diet, may be the best nutritional approach to treating insulin resistance.

Intake of dietary fat, particularly saturated fat, appears to be associated with insulin resistance in animals and humans and may predispose to the development of diabetes. It seems prudent at this time to advocate increased fiber consumption. Resistant starch or low GI diets may ultimately prove to have beneficial effects at some stage in the development of type 2 diabetes, but this remains controversial. Although simple sugars appear to cause insulin resistance in rats, adverse effects in humans have not been demonstrated conclusively. Future studies should use appropriate doses of these nutrients fed over moderate periods of time to populations presumed to be the most susceptible to their effects. These populations might be the young in the case of simple sugars and those with preexisting insulin resistance in the case of complex carbohydrate and fiber. Clear relationships may not emerge until it is possible to obtain a more accurate phenotype or even genotype of subjects because genetic heterogeneity likely underlies the heterogeneous response to these diets.

Studies relating specific foods to specific disease states may provide the most useful information for nutrition policy decisions. If the relationship between a nutrient and insulin sensitivity is to be examined, then specific measures of insulin action in the tissue that is likely to be affected or likely to be related to disease risk should be undertaken. Simply using insulin and glucose levels is unlikely to provide meaningful insights into these relationships. The relationships between diet and insulin action remain an important area for future investigation

PCOS DIET

Elena Miller

INSULIN Resistance Diet

Elena Miller

Pre-DIABETES Action Plan

Elena Miller

GUT Health Diet

Elena Miller